BACH FLOWER REMEDIES

REMEDIES

for Horses and Riders

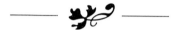

BACH FLOWER REMEDIES

for Horses and Riders

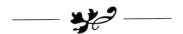

MARTIN J. SCOTT

with

Gael Mariani

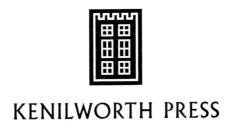

KENILWORTH PRESS

First published in Great Britain 2000 by
Kenilworth Press
Addington
Buckingham
MK18 2JR

British Library Cataloguing in Publication Data
A CIP record for this book is available from the British Library

ISBN 1-872082-25-5

Typeset in 11/13 Bembo
Illustrations by Carole Vincer
Typesetting and layout by Kenilworth Press
Printed and bound in Great Britain by
Hillman Printers (Frome) Ltd

DISCLAIMER

**This book is not to be used in place of veterinary
care and expertise.** No responsibility can be accepted by the
author, publishers or distributors of this book for the application
of any of the enclosed information in practice.

CONTENTS

Foreword *by Dr Trevor M. Cook*   7

Preface   9

Introduction – What are Bach Flower   11
    Remedies?

1   The Life and Work of Dr Edward Bach   17

2   The Bach Flower Remedies   24

3   The Horse   53

4   The Rider/Handler   64

5   Bach Flower Remedies in Practice   70

6   Case Studies   75

7   Helping Others   88

Conclusion   90

Useful Addresses   91

Index   93

*This book is dedicated to the memory of Chewbacca and Lady,
two very special and dear horses who are no longer with us and who are
sorely missed.*

FOREWORD

by

Dr Trevor M. Cook

As a former breeder and owner of thoroughbreds and having been involved with the Bach flower remedies during my career in complementary therapy, I was intrigued by this book by Martin Scott and Gael Mariani, which I understand is the first to specifically link the use of the remedies exclusively to horses and their owners and trainers.

I have always recognised the close bond between people and horses at the mental and emotional level, which makes the intrinsic properties of the Bach flower remedies even more relevant in this context. It is my view that whilst we may recognise physical differences in general, we do not always give animals credit for possessing individual mental, emotional and psychological characteristics, so I congratulate the authors of this book for focusing on this humane approach. It deserves to be read by anyone involved with horses, whether they be at stud, in the show ring, racehorses or for leisure riding.

Dr Trevor M. Cook, PhD, MSc, BSc,
DHom(Med), DIHom, HMD, NMD, FRSC, FHMA
Director, the British Institute of Homoeopathy
Former President of the Homoeopathic Medical Association (UK)
Co-founder of the British Association of Homoeopathic Veterinary Surgeons
Former supplier of animal health and nutrition products to HM The Queen

CAUTION

It must be mentioned here that this book is not to be used in place of veterinary care. If the horse is unwell, then the owner must call a veterinary surgeon to attend to the animal. If you fail to consult a vet in cases involving a serious medical condition, or in any way neglect your responsibilities as the horse's owner/keeper, you could be breaking the law. In the UK the Veterinary Surgeons' Act (1966) makes it illegal for any person who is not a veterinary surgeon to treat or advise on the treatment of any condition or disease of someone else's horse. American laws regarding these matters vary. Readers outside the UK are therefore advised to consult local sources for current regulations governing animal treatment and the use of natural remedies.

PREFACE

The purpose of this book is to demonstrate the striking effectiveness of Bach flower therapy for horses and their human counterparts. It is my desire to make the remedies accessible to anyone and everyone involved with horses at every level, and to help unlock the pleasures of equestrian sport and leisure for those suffering emotional barriers that hamper their enjoyment of their horse. The Bach flower remedies can make a real difference for anyone suffering difficulties in their riding, or in any other aspects of caring for their horse – whether the problem comes from themselves or the animal – and can help the many, many horses that suffer problems and pain related to the mind and emotions, whatever the cause might be.

For those readers new to the flower remedies, you will find it a fascinating new world – I hope I can do it justice and inspire you to make use of it. For those people already acquainted with Dr Bach's system, it is hoped that the book will fill in a few gaps, provide a fresh look, and maybe even enhance your use of the remedies so that you may continue to obtain maximum benefit from them. And although this is written very much for those involved with horses, we all have a life outside our particular interests and hobbies, with attendant fears, worries and stresses that can eat into our enjoyment of our chosen pastime. Let this book also be your guide to improving aspects of the emotions in general day-to-day living. A happier person overall makes a happier rider overall, and makes the horse happier too.

This therapy is so very simple to use, and so effective, that in truth it is a revolution waiting to happen. Though the remedies have lain relatively dormant for many years, the world about us and the way we think are changing fast. Perhaps the time has now come for Edward Bach's dream to be realised to its full extent?

Martin J. Scott

INTRODUCTION

What are Bach flower remedies?

Bach (pronounced 'batch') flower remedies have been with us for some seventy years, and as interest in complementary therapies in general increases worldwide, a growing number of people are coming to recognise their amazing power.

In the simplest terms, they are a collection of thirty-eight different liquid remedies, all derived entirely from nature and utterly pure in essence; they are simple to use and completely free of the side-effects that mar many of our conventional medicines. They are the work of one man, Dr Edward Bach (1886-1936), a person of extraordinary vision and genius whose dream it was to make it possible for the pure and innocent healing powers inherent in nature to benefit all mankind.

Whereas other forms of complementary therapy, for instance homoeopathy, are designed to work (primarily) directly on the body and the physical manifestations of illness, the Bach flowers are a system totally devoted to healing problems that stem from imbalances within the mind and emotions. Each individual remedy is geared to a specific, clearly defined, negative mental/emotional state and has the power, lifted from nature, to heal it. Between them they encompass the entire range of human, and for that matter animal, emotional experience, allowing us to treat all those states of fear, doubt, worry, anger, envy, gloom, etc., that hamper us throughout our lives and prevent us from being all we could be, and from living life to the full with the maximum of joy.

The impact of emotional negativity

Western society's conventional way of thinking all too often implies a dichotomy between the mind and the body, with the mind firmly classified as a second-class citizen. We often hear the phrase 'it's all in the mind' used to belittle, or even altogether dismiss, the importance of our emotional state. Many people adopt the hard-hearted attitude (and most of the blame here must go to the members of my own sex) that anyone suffering from emotional difficulties is being 'soft', a 'wimp'; that they can somehow be shamed out of it by being told: 'Come on – get a grip on yourself. Snap out of it!'

One might as well demand that we 'snap out of' a viral infection, or a wound, or a broken bone. Anyone who has ever suffered tension knows how much worse they feel when told to 'relax'; the same goes for people in depressive states when we demand that they 'cheer up'. It just does not work that way! Yet people persist with their blinkered attitudes. It is as though they are afraid of admitting to the importance of emotional pain, or worse, they attach a stigma of shame to it.

We need to think about negative mental and emotional states in a sensible down-to-earth way, the same way we would think about a cut finger or a strained ankle. Just as these temporary physical impairments prevent us from carrying out daily tasks such as opening a bottle, or walking from A to B, so emotional negativity often prevents people from participating fully and joyfully in life. And just like the finger and the ankle, it can be helped to heal itself from within so that the pain leaves and we are once again able to carry on with our business.

Imbalances in the mind and emotions happen to us all: that is a simple fact. The state of happiness that we all seek is an elusive and fragile thing indeed. It teeters on a knife-edge; it is like a highly tuned engine that may suddenly just start to run 'sick'; or a musical instrument that may slip into disharmony, a minute detunement of one string spoiling the whole sound. Just as these inanimate things can be adjusted back into harmony, we all have it in us to attain our emotional potential, our ideal emotional state, and we all have our individual notion of exactly what that state would be like. A very timid person would dream of becoming socially confident and outgoing, perhaps more able to stand up for themselves; a nervous person might try to imagine the day when they could face the world with courage and shake off those feelings of fear and doubt; a person tormented by irrational guilt might yearn for a lightening of the destructive millstone around their neck.

This picture of ourselves at our full emotional potential is what is known as the Higher Self, or Higher Personality. The corresponding instinctual Lower Self, or Lower Personality, is the product of emotional blockages – fear, worry, regret, shame, etc. – that prevent the virtues and qualities of the Higher Self from shining through. This blocked and relatively unhappy personality is the way a great many of us, most of us in fact, see ourselves reflected in everyday life. Occasionally we might get a glimpse of our Higher Self, maybe when we carry out some selfless act of generosity, or when we are able to rise above our worries, or genuinely laugh at our own misfortunes. But all too often that side of us is hidden behind the clouds. What the Bach flower remedies do is help dissolve those negative emotional blockages, allowing a lighter state, our emotional potential, to emerge. It is a simple idea – and that simplicity, which will be echoed time and again in this book, is the great strength and beauty of the Bach flower system of healing. We do not need to be trained doctors or psychiatrists or behaviourists to understand it; we require no special knowledge, skill or gift. We require only the ability to see in ourselves, or in another living being, the emotional blockage that is causing trouble, be it fear, sadness or whatever. Thus, the means to use the Bach flower remedies, and to gain real results from them, lie in everyone's hands – your hands.

Bach flower remedies in the horse world

How does all this translate into our interest in horses? The fact is that many people involved in the realm of horses and horse-riding suffer emotional blockages that hamper their ability to fulfil their goals, whether those goals be participating in high-level sport or merely enjoying a pleasant hack through the countryside. Every riding instructor sees scores of people plagued with nervous tension and lack of confidence. These problems may be evinced at one end of the scale by a little stiffness in the saddle, to outright terror and phobia at the other.

There are a great many possible sources of anxiety, frustration and worry in the equestrian world; and for those in emotionally vulnerable states there seems to be trouble lurking at every turn. For people just starting out, a horse is a big animal that may seem very intimidating. Early frights and spills, even minor ones, can be very off-putting. Frustration at perceived lack of improvement in our skills can lead to despondency; friendly competitiveness with our peers may carry an undertone of real rivalry and cause anger. As our bond with our beloved horse grows, there comes the risk of heartbreak should anything happen to it. As we get older, we tend to become more aware of what might happen to us should things go wrong! Basically, we are scared of getting hurt – and who can blame us for that? Many people who have been riding for years, or who come back to riding after, say, raising a family, suddenly find themselves troubled with fears and preoccupations that would never have occurred to them in the past. Of course, caution is always a good thing, especially in a pursuit like riding that can be fraught with potential danger. But on the other hand, the over-cautiousness that comes with fear and worry also brings with it many problems for riders and handlers.

The horse: the ultimate Bach flower patient?

Animals, too, suffer problems stemming from the mind and emotions, although these are overlooked or ignored with painful regularity by we humans. Those of us who look after animals with love and respect are highly aware that they experience a whole variety of moods and states, just as we do. They are not objects or machines that exist merely to be used by us in all the many ways we do use them – they are sentient and highly sensitive beings that respond to good treatment, and to love and care. Like us, they have emotional needs and are capable of thoughts and reasoning that we may not always be able to see but would be stupid to disregard. Who has not felt a melting of the heart when their pet came up to them and rubbed up against them affectionately; when a dog came up and buried its face lovingly in their lap; or when a horse rumbled its greeting as they walked into the stable-yard in the morning?

Working with horses and watching their behaviour is a constant source of pleasure. They are as finely and elegantly tuned in mind as they are in body; they are wonderfully, deeply intelligent and have incredible powers of lateral thinking, logic and memory to rival (and occasionally surpass!) our own. The downside is that with such a range of emotional and mental states at hand, they share not only in our human capacity for tremendous joy and satisfaction, but also in our lamentable tendency to fall into negative states of mind and mood. The list is a long one: horses may be prone to terror, stubbornness, foul temper, mischief, aggression, boredom, bad habits, loneliness, over-attachment, grief, self-pity, jealousy, resentment and much more. These negative moods, which can be brief and fleeting or sometimes of a semi-permanent nature, can play havoc with our dealings and relations with our horses, often turning what was once a pleasurable pastime into a living nightmare and reducing proud, confident owners into gibbering wrecks.

This is where the Bach flower remedies come in, helping us to treat our own reactions in such a way as to cope with the problems at hand. In the treatment of horses, once the right remedy or combination of remedies is chosen, the effect is rarely anything less than spectacular. Horses that were quite literally pining away have been restored to full emotional health over exceptionally short periods, while others that had become dangerously aggressive have come back to their old approachable selves in no time at all. For this reason I am always tempted to describe the horse as the ultimate Bach flower patient! They are so pure in soul, so uncluttered with emotional garbage, so open and honest about the way they feel, that their response to treatment is almost infallibly swift and long-lasting.

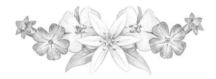

CHAPTER ONE

THE LIFE AND WORK OF
DR EDWARD BACH

From an early age Edward Bach was captivated by the beauty of nature, and he combined this with a great empathy for all living things that suffered. It was only natural that his life's path would be to help others, and in 1912, at the age of twenty-six, he qualified as a doctor.

Bach was a keen observer of people, a true humanist. Working in the wards of his London hospital, he would spend much time with patients, getting to know them and looking beyond their states of disease, at the individual people they were. At the same time, witnessing the treatment and recovery of these patients, he began to notice that, while some of them responded well to a given medicine and got better, others responded far less and their condition failed to improve. The inquiring young doctor wondered why this might be.

As time went by he began to note the different temperaments of the patients: there were those who were driven to despair and depression by their sickness; there were those who responded with anger and frustration; there were those who were fearful about what lay ahead of them; and those who were relatively philosophical and calm about their state of health. There seemed to be a correlation between the individual personalities of the patients, their state of mind, and the way they responded to treatment. Out of a group of people all given the same medicine for a particular ailment, those with a more positive outlook on their condition and on life in general would respond faster and better than those whose outlook was more pessimistic or defeatist. This latter group would respond weakly and were significantly more prone to going under.

Bach concluded from this that the personality of an individual held the key to their constitutional strength and was the overlooked factor in the treatment of disease. Thus he decided that if he could directly treat the emotional and mental state of his patients, he would be able to boost their resistance against illness and help make them better. He also believed that in many cases their negative outlook was the reason they had become ill in the first place. This conviction was to stay with him for the rest of his life, but at the same time it placed him at odds with the medical establishment to which he belonged. He felt that the medicine of his day lacked something vital; that there was more to the art of healing than met the eye of his peers.

Branching out into the field of immunology, Bach then had a major breakthrough. He had by now established seven basic temperamental/personality groups amongst his patients, and he experimented to find what each group had in common. He found the link in the intestinal bacteria, discovering that each personality group had its own specific bacterial characteristics. From each bacterial category in turn, Bach then created a group of seven vaccines, known as **nosodes**, and these medicines, administered by injection, proved to have a very potent curative effect on a whole range of chronic diseases. Before long, Bach was prescribing his nosodes to patients almost entirely on the basis of their personality type – and obtaining excellent results. He was becoming more and more convinced of the vital importance of the mental and emotional state to overall health.

But it bothered him that he was working with products derived from diseased tissues. Despite his success, he felt urged to look further. In 1919 he landed a job in a major homoeopathic hospital in London. Until this time he had never really come across homoeopathy, but on the eve of his first day at work there he stayed up reading for the first time the seminal book *The Organon of the Healing Art,* by Samuel Hahnemann, the creator of the homoeopathic system of medicine. He was enthralled. Homoeopathy stems from the principle that medical treatment should focus not on the disease, but rather on the individual patient. It employs medicinal remedies that are drawn from nature and are highly diluted so as to remove all traces of poisonous material, then energised, or 'potentised', to enhance the curative power. Administered orally and painlessly, they are deeply effective yet perfectly safe and gentle, causing no ill effect to the person treated.

These concepts struck a real chord in Dr Bach. Up until that point he had felt rather alone. At last, here was verification of many of his own ideas and beliefs! He immediately set about making up homoeopathic versions of his nosodes. To his delight, they were even more effective than before. He was now able to offer his medicines to patients in a manner that did away with the need for the hypodermic needle. But even more importantly, he had taken a major step away from using noxious substances as medicine.

As his work went on, he found himself observing people more and more, both in his clinic and during his hours of leisure. He became increasingly aware that it was possible to fit people's personality types into certain categories: the lonely, the oversensitive, the anxious, the domineering, and so on. And, fired as he was by his discovery of homoeopathy with its pure and gentle ways, he became more and more enthused with the notion of finding a totally unadulterated, harmless yet powerful treatment that could profoundly affect the blockages of the personality, the negative emotional states that he could see in people. He knew that in order to achieve this goal he would have to look beyond even homoeopathy, going right back to grass roots, as it were, and the healing forces of his beloved Nature.

He started experimenting, and soon discovered four plants that had remarkably similar curative properties to four of his own nosodes. The plants were Star of Bethlehem *(Ornithogalum umbellatum)*, Mimulus *(Mimulus guttatus)*, Impatiens *(Impatiens glandulifera)*, and Clematis *(Clematis vitalba)*. If it were possible to replace four of the nosodes, it must be possible to go further. This was now Bach's single-minded aim.

At this point he felt that his involvement with conventional medicine was finished. By 1930 he was running his own lucrative practice in London's prestigious Harley Street; but, spurred on by his initial findings, he packed his bags and set off on what amounted to a 'pilgrimage' of discovery, that was to take up every waking moment from then until the day he died.

Building on his earlier observation of his patients by continued study of people around him, Bach came up with seven distinct categories of negative mental/emotional states. These were:

1.   FEAR

2.   UNCERTAINTY

3.   LACK OF INTEREST IN PRESENT CIRCUMSTANCES

4.   LONELINESS

5.   OVERSENSITIVITY TO IDEAS AND INFLUENCES

6.   DESPONDENCY AND DESPAIR

7.   OVERCONCERN FOR THE WELFARE OF OTHERS

Subdividing these seven, he identified thirty-eight specific negative states of mind, each with its own positive-potential counterpart, that between them spanned the entire spectrum of all our emotional experience: that is, every undesirable mood, character trait and emotion that it is possible for mankind to experience. His ambition was to find thirty-eight remedies in all, one for each of these states, and create a whole new system of healing that would act directly where it mattered, healing away painful and destructive blockages to create a better and happier life for all who used it.

The discovery of the remedies

Living something of a nomadic existence, Bach travelled all around England and Wales. He spent much time walking in remote country areas where wild flowers grew in abundance; and he drew on ancient herbal wisdom, his own intuition and endless experimentation to discover more plants to add to his new system. He worked tirelessly, also travelling to other countries in his quest before returning to England and settling down in what was to be his last home, Mount Vernon, in the Oxfordshire countryside. After six long years of hard work, he had completed his search. He now had thirty-seven plant-derived remedies and a thirty-eighth that was prepared from a special source of spring water.

Bach adopted a method of 'potentising' which differed from homoeopathy in that he used heat to extract the beneficial potential from each natural raw material, either by boiling up the petals and buds, or leaving them to infuse in the sunlight. To preserve the delicate remedy liquid, it was diluted in mild brandy; then it was put into small amber-glass dropper bottles, ready for use. As he had intended, each remedy was specifically indicated to heal a particular type of mental/emotional ill. They could be combined together, without clashing or interfering, in order to create tailor-made prescriptions to fit any individual case. And because they were so natural and free of any kind of toxic content, they could be used without any fear of side-effects and alongside any other form of medication.

To Bach, his collection of remedies was a self-contained and complete system. As they covered between them every possible permutation of our emotional range, there was no need to add more remedies to the list – unlike homoeopathy, for instance, which has thousands. He felt he had completed his life's work and now concentrated on teaching his findings to others, lay people and health professionals alike.

In 1936, on his fiftieth birthday, he announced his new system to the public. Shortly afterwards, in November of that year, he finally allowed himself to give in to the cancer that had been diagnosed many years earlier. Before he died, he entrusted the future of his remedies to his companions and followers. He specified that the Bach flower system be left unchanged in the future, that it be taught to successive generations just as he had intended it.

Simplicity was, is, and always will be, the keyword of the Bach flower remedies. Bach's vision was that they should be accessible to everyone. He insisted that they must be affordable, so that every family, every home, could have a set. No medical training was necessary to understand them; there was no need to wrestle with complex scientific theories or plough through enormous volumes of text. While the Bach flower system was capable of so much and went to the very root of disease, it was clear and simple enough to be understood by everyone.

How do the remedies work?

There is a short answer to this question, and there is a long answer. The short answer is that nobody really knows how the Bach remedies work. Those of us who have seen them work know that they do so most effectively. To an extent, that is all one should need to say about them. After all, we should not forget that much of modern medicine, having its origins in ancient herbalism, is derived from plants. The curative properties of nature have been known ever since the first humans began discovering, most likely by trial and error as well as following the example of animals, which berries and leaves and bark would harm you when eaten, and which ones would make you better. Much is taken for granted, not everything can be explained in simple biochemical terms. It is simply down to our past collective experience.

That seems to be good enough for those of us who trust in conventional medicine, i.e. virtually all of us. But for the detractors of complementary medicine, the apparent gaps in our knowledge present a convenient target. It is often said of homoeopathy, for example, that with the 'mother tincture', the raw material of the remedy, diluted away literally to nothing, it is not possible that there could be any curative power in the finished tablet or liquid. Similarly, the active medicine in the Bach flower remedies actually contains none of the original plant solids from which it is derived. So what, we might ask, is going on inside us when we take a Bach flower remedy?

We are dealing here with something so subtle, so sophisticated, that we have not yet been able to comprehend it fully. The Bach remedies are infused in water, and as the science of molecular chemistry progresses, it is believed that the capacity of water to retain an imprint, a signature or memory, is at the heart of how these complementary methods work. It is only recently that we have started to learn how to measure the changes that occur in the water at a sub-molecular level when the healing vibrations of the plant material are transferred into it via the potentisation procedure, and we do know that changes occur. We may further speculate that the water-borne remedy, carrying with it the imprinted signature of the healing plant, releases vibrations into our being that harmonise with our Higher Self or Higher Personality, allowing the blockages to vanish and the positive potential locked inside to flood through us — as Bach envisaged, a 'drawing down' of cleansing power through our entire body and soul that restores us to a positive emotional state and subsequently a positive physical state.

Given the speed with which science continually peels back the layers of the unknown, we can surely expect that sooner or later an explanation will come forth that should prove satisfactory to even the most cynical disbeliever.

In the meantime, it should not really be of any great importance to us that we have yet to understand the exact workings of these things. Samuel Hahnemann, when he was developing his homoeopathic system, actually had no interest at all in how it might work; he was simply aware that it did, and he got on with the task of perfecting it. We have the same situation here with regard to the Bach flower remedies. It is foolish to refuse to accept something simply because we do not know how it works, even more so when we only have to observe it to see that it does. How many of us understand fully the mechanics of what happens when we press down the accelerator pedal in our car? We don't need to know. We only need to know that the car will go faster. So we press the pedal down, the car goes faster, and we are satisfied with the result. Taking a broader view, there are many things in the world and the universe around us that we do not yet understand. What is fire? We know how to make it and how to put it out – but we do not know what it is. What is life itself, this fundamental, invisible force that animates our fleshly bodies? Again, we know how to propagate it, and we certainly have demonstrated quite a talent for extinguishing it. But do we know for sure what it is?

To those detractors who argue that the Bach flower remedies rely entirely on placebo effect, I would point out the title and subject matter of this book! The fact that the flower remedies, along with many other forms of complementary therapy, work on animals is really the absolute proof of their efficacy and blows away all cynical objections. Placebos are often used in treating humans – they are a long-standing tool in the conventional medical kitbag – and it has been demonstrated that when a person is convinced they can get better, they very often do. This is a simple truth, and in fact it, along with its converse – that a person convinced they will get worse, will get worse – is part of the philosophy behind the Bach flower remedies. But animals do not play such mind games, and the placebo effect is an irrelevance where they are concerned. They either get better, or they do not. They are either distraught, or they are calm. And so on. To suggest otherwise would be ridiculous – it would be to imply that when your horse sees you coming with a bottle of flower remedy to drip into his water bucket, he thinks to himself: 'Oh yes; that must be because the blacksmith's coming on Wednesday and they want me on my best behaviour.'

In short, I feel confident that we can leave aside complex scientific theories and explanations as to how the remedies work. Our task is simply to assure ourselves that they do, and to endeavour to use them to help ourselves and others, whilst leaving the technical matters, which at the end of the day are little more than a matter of curiosity, to those best equipped to deal with them. Dr Bach would have approved of this attitude, and what was good enough for Dr Bach should be good enough for us!

In the next chapter we begin to look in detail at the remedies he developed, one by one.

CHAPTER TWO

THE BACH FLOWER REMEDIES

As mentioned earlier, Dr Bach's thirty-eight remedies are divided into seven distinct groups. Some practitioners have more or less done away with the group headings, and regard the remedies as one big group that can be listed alphabetically. While this is fine, in my opinion looking at the remedies under their original seven category titles serves to give a better feel for them and is also an aid to memory. Thirty-eight remedies might not seem a lot at first glance, but it is a fair amount to remember!

As this book is dealing specifically with matters related to the horse and rider, some of the following remedies will be more widely indicated and more useful than others. While every remedy will be examined in these pages, I shall go into certain ones in greater depth. Those that are particularly well suited to typical horse-and-rider scenarios are indicated with an asterisk ✩.

1. Fear

We tend to think of fear simply as fear. But in this group there are five distinct angles on the concept of fear. To pick the right remedy for a person – or animal – that is in some way afraid, we need to look closely at each description and see which one matches the closest. The five remedies under this heading are Rock Rose, Mimulus, Cherry Plum, Aspen and Red Chestnut.

ROCK ROSE ✩ *Helianthemum nummularium*

Dr Bach designated Rock Rose to treat acute states of extreme fear and terror, and their aftermath. It is for when we feel as though we are in great danger. The mind races uncontrollably, the heart pounds, and there is the irresistible urge to run away from whatever thing or situation is posing such a terrifying threat. There may be fear of death or mutilation. It is the remedy for accidents, or for sudden severe illness that gives rise to great terror.

Rock Rose would also be indicated in cases where the danger is not so real, but nonetheless provokes a terrified reaction. For instance, many people suffer panic-attacks for all kinds of reasons: going to the dentist is a classic example, or having an injection; these have been known to reduce otherwise stoic and brave people into quivering jellies! In horse-riding it is a first-line remedy, very useful indeed for calming the nerves and very fast-acting. Nervous beginners, people who have had accidents and are afraid of getting back into riding as their minds are full of images of pain and fright, or riders who are just generally nervous, would all benefit from the remedy. The goal of the remedy is to bring out the positive potential of inner courage, to achieve heroic self-transcendence.

Similarly horses, as flight/prey animals, often react to stimuli with terror and instinctively want to run away. Rock Rose is the remedy for this.

MIMULUS ✩ *Mimulus guttatus*

The Mimulus remedy deals with a less pressing, less acute, everyday state of fear. A person in need of Mimulus would be anxious about something specific, whether it be a situation they have to face, something they have to do, or a person they have to meet. Driving tests, exams, public appearances, first dates, are all potentially Mimulus situations. Of course, if these things caused real horror and trembling, Rock Rose could be used instead or in addition.

There is generally an anticipatory element in Mimulus fear, with a refusal to think about some undesirable thing, something dreaded. There are some people who are in a near-constant Mimulus state. They are nervous of any little thing, any situation that calls for them to push themselves. Very timid and retiring people, shy children, or those tending towards weakness of character who are nervy and fearful, would all benefit from the remedy.

Because it is indicated for less acute states of fear than Rock Rose, it works more slowly, building up one's courage over a period of a few days or weeks. If one had to face up to some slightly scary event, such as a competitive riding event, and was feeling a sense of nervous anticipation (as is normal), it would be a good idea to start taking Mimulus ten days to two weeks before the dreaded day.

CHERRY PLUM 🟇 *Prunus cerasifera*

Cherry Plum, despite its pretty name, deals with some of the most frightening mental/emotional states around. In the Cherry Plum state, the mind has fallen out of balance; the person feels crazed, with thoughts and impulses popping up from the dark recesses of the imagination that may seem shocking, weird and disturbing in nature.

Taken to extremes, this mental state can lead to reckless, impulsive and risky behaviour; or even worse, may involve irrational and powerful desires to do harm either to others or to oneself. Such wild impulses can be so strong as actually to take over and control our conduct. Many crimes, murders and suicides are committed by people in a Cherry Plum state. The loss of control over the rational mind is very frightening, and the sufferer struggles to suppress the terrifying thought-content and to restore balance and calm. This is what the remedy helps to do.

Similarly, an animal that has turned savage and dangerous as a result of its fear, perhaps due to pain or ill-treatment, can be calmed with the remedy. The great benefit here is that no physical contact with the animal would be necessary – if it can be contained in an enclosure or stable, all that is needed is a small amount of drinking water with a few drops of remedy added. However furious and tormented the animal, sooner or later it must drink, effectively treating itself while we watch from a safe distance. In severe cases, it would be advisable to call the vet, and quickly.

There are, thankfully, lighter shades of the Cherry Plum state. These would be milder cases where unwanted, irrational thoughts are exerting pressure on the mind. Panicky states, for example. If a person is sitting on the back of a horse and their mind's eye is constantly throwing at them images of falling off, of death and carnage, of the horse suddenly rearing up and hurling them to the ground, Cherry Plum is definitely indicated, perhaps in conjunction with Rock Rose. In fact, the two are both ingredients of the famous Bach **Rescue Remedy**, which is very often used as a general nerve-soother. (We will be looking in depth at Rescue Remedy later in the book.)

ASPEN *Populus tremula*

Those in need of Aspen are fearful and afraid, even to the point of trembling, and their state may carry on for a long time. But what marks this remedy is that the fear cannot be explained, cannot be attributed to anything in particular. In the Aspen state we cannot feel safe; we are as if haunted. Sometimes a fearful state that might initially seem to stem from something definite and specific actually turns out to be an Aspen state. For example, a person who is very seriously ill and at risk of death may be extremely afraid – but if the object of their fear is the great unknown, perhaps with a metaphysical slant, they are in need of this remedy.

Animals are often seen slinking about nervously before a storm. They can sense in the air that something is afoot, something is wrong, something is about to happen. But what? They are not quite sure, and therein lies the true nature of their fear. This element of mystery is the key to identifying the Aspen fear state.

RED CHESTNUT *Aesculus carnea*

This final remedy under the heading FEAR deals with a very particular type of fear: a fear for the well-being of others. In the Red Chestnut state we are constantly worried that someone close to us is in danger, and our mind is flooded with images of all that might befall them. Often, the loved one is far out of reach and the sense of powerlessness only compounds our worry that some awful accident is going to take place. This very distressing, yet frequently unwarranted, fear is often experienced by parents worried about their children when they are out of sight.

The goal of the treatment is not to prevent people from caring about each other's welfare, but rather to allow them to develop the ability to step back, consider that their fear may not be justified, and lessen their own nervousness and agitation.

What should always be borne in mind is that many of the emotional states that can be treated with Bach flower remedies are actually perfectly normal, and there is often no harm in experiencing them – in fact it is necessary to experience them to some degree. Here, with the Red Chestnut state, it is only right that we should be concerned about a loved one, whether it be our child out playing with friends, our partner or spouse travelling by plane, or our horse ten miles away at a livery stable. It is part of love, and part of life, to care about each other, and a person who is completely relaxed and unconcerned about the plight of those around him would come over as an unfeeling egocentric. But when emotions become too entrenched or distracting, that is when they need to be addressed, or else they can become a real problem – an emotional cancer eating away at our reserves of energy.

2. Uncertainty

There are six remedies in this category: Cerato, Scleranthus, Gentian, Gorse, Hornbeam and Wild Oat.

CERATO ✩ *Ceratostigma willmottiana*

Cerato is a healing flower for those of us who are hesitant and low in confidence. Such people have a problem trusting their own decisions and instead are overly reliant on the judgement and opinions of others, forever asking questions: 'How should I do this?'; 'What would you do in my position?' Therefore it is all but impossible for them to take charge of a situation or exert any authority. The problems a person in the Cerato state faces when dealing with animals, particularly big animals like horses, for instance, are quite plain, as they are incapable of asserting themselves – hence unable to gain the animal's respect in those situations when it might be required.

In everyday life, Cerato types will tend to be followers – they follow fashions, opinion-leaders, trends of various sorts. Shyness is a common trait. What people in this state need is a boost of confidence that would help release their inner wisdom, allow them to listen to their intuition and come to think independently.

SCLERANTHUS *Scleranthus annuus*

In the Scleranthus state, uncertainty is expressed in the sufferer's problems with regard to keeping a steady mind, for instance in decision-making. This would be the sort of person who simply cannot decide whether to travel to place A or place B for their vacation and will sit with a brochure in each hand, staring first at one and then at the other; they will decide on option A and start making arrangements for that, then suddenly change their mind and settle on option B, and will change their mind back and forth any number of times. Finally, having travelled to place B and sitting in their hotel room, their thoughts will start turning to what it would have been like to have gone to place A instead... And so, from this rut of indecision arises a state of chronic dissatisfaction, restlessness and mental disturbance. Left untreated, this can develop into lethargy and depression, or extreme agitation and ultimately even nervous breakdown.

Often thought of exclusively as a remedy for indecisiveness and hesitation, Scleranthus is actually indicated for the wider area of vacillation. Wherever there is a swaying of the mind, or an unsettled, jumpy, fluctuating state, Scleranthus can be of service. Very erratic behaviour in animals, with constant switching of attention from one thing to another, may indicate the need for this remedy.

GENTIAN✯ *Gentianella amarella*

Someone in a negative Gentian state of mind feels uncertain in that they do not trust their own capabilities. They are uncertain of themselves, uncertain that things will ever go right for them. When faced with difficulties in life they may feel that fate is against them; rather than press on and try to have faith in themselves and the future, they will tend instead to shrug their shoulders and give up. The remedy helps restore the lacking faith and optimism, and reinforces the will so that problems can be tackled, difficulties fought through.

An obvious use of the remedy would be for people learning the ropes of riding. Maybe it is proving more demanding, more difficult than they had first thought when they put their name down for lessons; maybe they are allowing the almost inevitable early setbacks and disappointments to get to them. When they start showing signs of flagging and talk of perhaps giving up, the benefits of Gentian are needed. After all, everyone has problems when they first embark upon a new pursuit – and this applies not only to equestrian sports but to every activity, every realm of interest known to us – and in many cases people have given up the struggle who might have gone on to great things. Faith, optimism and confidence were the virtues lacking: the very things that the remedy helps to bring out of us.

The positive Gentian state is reflected in the old story about the Scottish chieftain Robert the Bruce, who, lying low and feeling

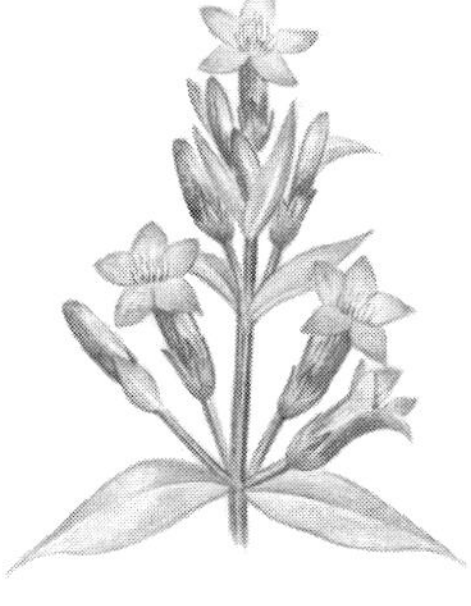

despondent and pessimistic after a defeat at the hands of the English, saw a spider trying to climb up a slippery vertical surface. It failed at first – but, undeterred, tried and tried until it eventually succeeded and was able to make its web. Inspired by this, the Bruce adopted the motto: 'If at first you don't succeed, try, try again!'

GORSE ✩ *Ulex europaeus*

In the Gorse state of mind we feel there is just no hope. It is a state of uncertainty that borders on despair; there is great resignation and apathy. It is common among the very sick, for instance in terminal illness where there seems to be no light at the end of the tunnel and no point in resisting one's fate. It is a sense of all-pervading pessimism and defeatism.

If we think back to Dr Bach's observations of his patients, one of the things that led him to develop his ideas was the way that people in such a negative state would be especially prone to succumbing to their illness, while the more optimistic patients had a better chance. Animals are just the same. When physical illness strikes, the spirits will sag – and it can be a very dangerous state when the animal has, in effect, lost the will to live.★ This is not ascribing human characteristics to our furry friends; to illustrate the potential benefit of Gorse, experience has shown that even plants, for instance young seedlings that were weak, wilting and in danger of dying, have grown stronger and survived when fed a small amount of the remedy. This is not as incredible as it might seem, if we stop to think about it for a moment. Every living thing has the potential to grow and be strong, just as it has the potential to grow weak, fall ill and die. Humans have the ability to analyse their emotional and physical states, to put words to them, in a way that, as far as we know, the other living species do not – but however we choose to envisage them or describe them, the forces at work that dictate strength or weakness, life or death, are the same whether the subject be a person or a tiny plant. It is very easily done, but we should not forget our place in the great natural scheme of things!

Gorse is also a good remedy for situations of bereavement, where grief is very bitter and there is a nihilistic sense of 'What's the point of anything any more?' It works to lift the spirits, making it possible to look to the future and say with restored certainty: 'It's going to be all right!'

★In cases of physical illness afflicting your horse, you should always consult your vet. The Bach flower remedies are **not** intended as a replacement for veterinary medical care.

HORNBEAM ✵ *Carpinus betulus*

Hornbeam is the remedy that addresses the so-called 'Monday-morning feeling'. Such a state is just another angle on the idea of uncertainty, in that we are lacking the power in our mind, willpower if you like, to see us through our tasks. Duties and chores will stretch out in front of us like a prison sentence. Those of us in the horsey world are all too aware of how awful and depressing a long winter of muddy paddocks, damp tack, wet rugs and constant mucking out can be. There are times when it is extremely hard to muster the mental energy to face our tasks. Our minds can go hazy and we tend to procrastinate. If we catch ourselves thinking 'I'll do this later on; I just cannot be bothered to do it now…', we have entered the Hornbeam state.

People who allow this kind of state to go on can fall into a chronic lethargy that is like a mild depression. Hornbeam is very good for restoring the missing spark, and can help renew concentration and focus.

WILD OAT *Bromus ramosus*

The Wild Oat type is a person with a real need to push themselves, to develop themselves; they have a true 'hunger' and innate desire to achieve something in their lives. The problem is, they have trouble deciding what their calling is and how they are going to express their talents. It is often the case that they are not consciously fully aware of these desires and needs, and are troubled by a vague sense of boredom and frustration. With the inner urge for growth stifled and repressed in this way, the emotions may veer towards joylessness and depression. Nothing quite satisfies them; they scratch around in life, moving from phase to phase, and while they may show talent and ability in different areas, they are insufficiently motivated to go into anything in any depth.

Young riders who show a lot of natural aptitude, yet are not ambitious enough or committed enough to exploit that talent, might benefit from Wild Oat. The remedy rekindles incentive, and those who benefit from it rapidly gain a great sense of satisfaction, knowing that they have a way of channelling their abilities constructively.

The other aspect of the Wild Oat state is its occasional tendency to come on when we are tired, overworked, or too one-sidedly focused on a particular goal. Someone training hard for a competition or examination could be prone to this temporary state, losing motivation and joy of progress. In such a case it could be that other remedies, Hornbeam for instance, would be needed in addition to Wild Oat.

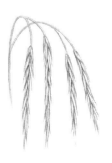

3. Lack of interest in present circumstances

The mental/emotional states here relate to a disinterest in our environment, the people and situations around us – either due to feeling disconnected from the world or feeling unmotivated to join in. There are seven remedies in this group: these are Clematis, Honeysuckle, Wild Rose, Olive, White Chestnut, Mustard and Chestnut Bud.

CLEMATIS *Clematis vitalba*

In the Clematis state, the lights are on, but nobody is home. The state is one of dreaminess, listlessness, lack of alertness. People who have fallen into this mental state are disconnected from the here and now and live in a world of their own, a dream-world. They can feel detached from the physical world and their own bodies, and the world about them holds little or no interest. They are very easily distracted, prone to falling into reverie while at work or school, and will be regarded as 'dreamers'. Romantic or escapist fantasies are often played out in their minds, and their imagination becomes the internal cinema screen to which they retreat.

Riding instructors will be familiar with the sight of the little boy or girl in their class group who is always last in line and sits gazing into space while their pony plods along more or less unguided! The chances are that they are like this most of the time, always day-dreaming and not quite 'there'. Clematis would be of use in giving a new focus and increased powers of alertness and concentration.

HONEYSUCKLE ✳ *Lonicera caprifolium*

This is a great remedy for home-sickness, nostalgia and sadness relating to something lost or something left behind. These are states of detachment from the world around, where the mind is dwelling excessively in the past. It is a sad state, and those experiencing it may feel that they will never again be able to find happiness. It is of much use in situations of bereavement, not just at the time but for a long time, perhaps years, afterwards, when we find ourselves recalling the good times we have had and thinking they are lost and gone forever. Many people who have lost a favourite horse, even though they might have found another that they dearly love, would benefit from Honeysuckle. Typically they find themselves overly saddened by thoughts of the past, which could be evoked by riding through an old haunt, the sight of an old feed bucket, a disused saddle or an empty stable.

Horses, too, suffer from Honeysuckle states when they lose a companion, or when they are moved to a new home, in which latter case the remedy is well backed up with **Walnut** for the change of surroundings. Giving them this remedy allows them some freedom from their sorrow and boosts their interest in their present surroundings.

WILD ROSE✶ *Rosa canina*

The Wild Rose state may arise when the 'slings and arrows of outrageous fortune' have become too much to bear. These people have struggled against the hardships of life to a point where their will is broken and they retreat into a resigned state of apathy. They are looking for a safe corner within themselves, where they will feel less threatened.

Animals that fall into this emotional/mental state are beyond fear, beyond rebellion. They have disappeared into themselves and become totally passive. Horses, being particularly sensitive creatures, can become like this after a terrible shock, for instance after years of cruelty or maltreatment. They may have gone through a phase initially where they reacted with terror or aggression; but as time passes, their mental reserves and their pride are so depleted that this pitiful 'zombiefied' state is all that remains. In cases where past traumas have inflicted terrible mental scars, the remedy could be given alongside **Star of Bethlehem**. Treatment may be long-term if trauma has gone very deep, but gradually the remedy allows the vital spark to return, allowing for a renewal of trust and happiness.

OLIVE✶ *Olea europoea*

Olive comes into play in situations of intense fatigue. It is a state that we all know: that feeling that we have reached the end of our tether, that we simply cannot go on. Nothing seems to matter any more, and the need to flop into bed is foremost in our minds. Weariness and exhaustion seem to have permeated every corner of mind and body. The state could come on at the end of an arduous task, such as punishing physical labour. I have used it on myself when absolutely worn out after a day's hay-making in the hot sun. The remedy really does have a revitalising quality. It refreshes mind and body, giving the feeling that the depleted reserves of energy are recharged.

Animals suffering heatstroke may also benefit from being given Olive, in more severe cases perhaps in conjunction with **Rescue Remedy**. Our big Rottweiler dog, Mungo, who dislikes the heat at the best of times, overdid things on a very warm day and was in a state of near-collapse; Olive brought him back to life very quickly. After a hard day's cross-country or endurance riding, after which horse and rider may be very tired, both could most certainly benefit from this remedy.

People can suffer chronically from an Olive state. Long-term physical weakness then affects the emotions. Appearing burnt-out, such people cannot get excited about anything, even things which previously brought them great joy. They may sink into sadness, depression, apathy and a sense of futility. Faced with someone in this state, the responsible practitioner should encourage them to take medical advice if they have not already done so. Chronic fatigue of this kind may have many causes; it might be worth considering dietary issues such as iron deficiency. The same applies to horses. If your horse appears constantly tired and listless, certain tests might be required and the vet should be consulted. Anaemia, worm infestation or a range of other factors may come into play. If the horse receives the all-clear from the vet, Olive will be of great use to help stimulate that lost energy. It could also be used alongside any other medication that the vet prescribes, to boost recovery. Again, such is the practical, flexible simplicity of the Bach remedies.

WHITE CHESTNUT *Aesculus hippocastanum*

This is the remedy for constant preoccupation. In this kind of mental/emotional state we are forever thinking about matters, forever reflecting, analysing, replaying events and dialogue in our mind. The problem comes when we find we cannot switch off, and those thoughts become an unwanted swirl that may take over completely, possibly keeping us awake at night and interfering with our routine, our work, our whole life. In fact this sort of constant worrisome preoccupation can, if left untreated, lead to the development of physical ailments such as migraine.

A person in such a state finds it hard to relax, and will often tend to be tense in their muscles. For riders this is an undesirable trait. Horses are very quick to pick up on negative body-language, and nervous tension is easily transmitted to the horse instead of the positive, confident signals we should be sending out. White Chestnut helps us to release the pressure of constant thoughts, washing away the tendency to introspection and setting the mind free.

MUSTARD *Sinapis arvensis*

If you feel gloomy, miserable, cut off from life and very depressed, yet there is no apparent reason for these feelings, Mustard is the remedy indicated.

It is the inexplicability of the negative emotional state that differentiates it from other 'depressed' states; in **Gentian** we have a particular reason for feeling down, such as having lost our job or suffering some setback or failure. In **Gorse** or **Sweet Chestnut** we are able to express our gloom verbally. But in Mustard we don't really know what is going on – it is as if a black cloud had settled upon us from nowhere, like a total eclipse of the emotions. There are no obvious connections to the rest of our life's affairs. We need to ask ourselves whether perhaps there is something we are not revealing to ourselves. Is there some repressed undercurrent of sadness? (Think of **Star of Bethlehem**, **Agrimony**.) Are we maybe tired or worn out? (Think of **Hornbeam**, **Olive**, **Wild Oat**.) If the answer to these questions is a definite no, consider Mustard.

The remedy dispels gloom, and disperses the black cloud overhead. We will be able to embrace those times in our life when we feel existentially 'down', taking the bad with the good and not allowing the negative side to take us over. Inner tranquillity and serenity are made possible, with a renewed enjoyment of life. The benefits of achieving such positive potential will be seen in every activity we undertake, whereas left untreated, the Mustard state will detract from all that we do.

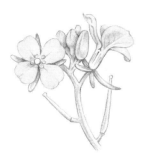

CHESTNUT BUD ✲ *Aesculus hippocastanum*

This remedy comes from the same Chestnut tree that provides the essence for the White Chestnut remedy. The latter is drawn from the tree's flowers, whereas this remedy, as the name would suggest, is prepared from the buds.

The Chestnut Bud state is one of restlessness, where the mind is not firmly rooted in the here and now. It treats tendencies to distraction, absent-mindedness and the kind of fidgety, unsettled mental behaviour that can be observed in the young and/or immature – the 'budding'. Problems with concentration and learning with regard to schoolwork have been helped using this remedy. In general life, people showing signs of the Chestnut Bud state may often fail to learn the lessons of their experience; instead of taking note of their mistakes and deriving wisdom from them, they tend to repeat the same errors over and over again, even when they suffer each time they do it.

People who repeatedly fail in business, or who continually misjudge human nature and allow themselves to be taken advantage of (see also **Centaury**), would in a great many cases benefit from Chestnut Bud. People who keep making mistakes by buying horses that are unsuitable for them, for instance owning a series of highly-strung Arabs when what they need is a sensible old 'school-master', would be another example.

Animals who are overly impulsive and spontaneous in their behaviour, particularly younger animals with huge reserves of energy, may be showing signs of a Chestnut Bud state. Horses that repeatedly barge despite being rebuked, are too easily distracted from their training, or need to think more carefully about what they are doing, could be helped with the remedy.

4. Loneliness

When we think of the term 'lonely' we tend to look at it in just one way: the image of a person left alone and longing for some company or love that has been taken away from them, for instance the imposed state we suffer after a marriage separation, or a bereavement. Dr Bach classified three different types of loneliness, and the states here deal more with aspects of the personality, or conscious steps taken, that distance us from others – hence causing emotional negativity, since deep down we want to be part of the world, interacting with our fellows. The three remedies in this group are: Water Violet, Impatiens and Heather.

WATER VIOLET *Hottonia palustris*

In this state, the person's desire for distance, seclusion from others' rests on their feeling that they are superior to those others. Hence they are unwilling to associate with them or descend to what they see as a lower level. A snobbish, narcissistic exterior hides a vulnerable, lonely inner core. The remedy helps to promote openness and acceptance of others and the ability to let go of concepts of social, intellectual or aesthetic hierarchy. An excellent remedy for 'spoilt brat syndrome' – if, that is, one could persuade the individual to look objectively at himself!

In my experience, the remedy is not one generally indicated for horses or other animals. Horses are herd animals and in general, brief quarrels and skirmishes notwithstanding, derive comfort and reassurance from each other's presence; a horse that deliberately keeps itself apart from the rest might be ill or in pain, and should be given a medical check.

It has sometimes been suggested that many cats, with their often disdainful, aloof bearing, would benefit from the remedy. But the error of this suggestion lies in the fact that cats are not suffering from being like this. Quite the opposite, in fact – it is a perfectly natural state for them. They are quite genuinely self-reliant creatures, able to be alone without being lonely, who can generally take us or leave us. They enjoy a certain degree of attention from us, but when they become bored with that and have obtained what they wanted from us, they happily go back to just being cats, a role they fill to perfection and evidently enjoy. There is sometimes a fine line between wishing to help alleviate emotional suffering in animals, and wishing to shape their behaviour to fit our own preferences – in this case wanting the cat to be our constant faithful companion the way a dog might be. This is an example of how the Bach flower remedies might be misunderstood by people who misinterpret the animal mind. In practice, however, this poses absolutely no threat to the animal, as the remedy, being prescribed for a perceived 'problem' that is simply the animal's natural state, would just not have any effect. If it could we would be imposing our will on the animal and perverting its innate characteristics in order to massage our own ego, which goes against all nature and the whole ethos of the Bach flower remedies.

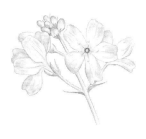

IMPATIENS ✩ *Impatiens glandulifera*

Impatiens is easily remembered as the remedy for impatience. In this emotional state, we are driven apart from others by our sense of being held back by them. It is an urgent, intolerant state of mind in which we can be irritable towards others. Very often it can be seen in the workplace, where some people will have a faster pace than others – perhaps those with more experience. But rather than use their superior skills, knowledge, experience, or whatever the case may be, to help and guide the slower ones, the efficient ones tend to feel tense and frustrated. As a result they are people who prefer to work on their own, where they are not hampered by having to make compromises for others. But where this is not an option and people are forced to work in a team, tempers can quickly fray.

Impatiens types may feel forced to set themselves up as leaders – not in the ambitious, power-hungry **Vine** sense (see later), but simply in order to 'get things done'. In doing so they may appear ruthless, insensitive and intimidating. In the office scenario, the Impatiens state is partly responsible for the rising incidence of what journalists call 'desk rage', namely angry outbursts between colleagues working in a highly stressed, competitive environment.

Any collective or team activity can be rapidly spoilt by the presence of an Impatiens type of person. In riding, some instructors are seen to lapse into the state when frustrated by a slow-learning or nervous pupil.

We have all experienced annoyance and frustration when working with animals. We are often under pressure to get things done; there might be a dozen lots of feed to mix, various other tasks to attend to, things to clean or repair. It might be getting dark and we feel we are working against the clock; maybe we have families at home waiting to be fed. In this state we can become rather snappy and bossy with our animals when they are slow to respond to our wishes. The horse that adamantly insists on having a last munch at the grass before it will come to us to be boxed for the night can really wind us up and provoke extreme frustration. Likewise the horse that won't get out of the way when we want to pass by with a bundle of hay for it. It can seem as though they are doing these things on purpose, deliberately holding us up just to annoy us. Of course, this is not the case; it is our perception that is at fault. It is the same as when we are in a hurry to get somewhere by car and it seems as though the other motorists on the road are conspiring to drive slowly just to hold us back! This is what gives rise to the phenomenon of 'road rage', the wheeled version of 'desk rage'.

Impatiens is the remedy (sometimes along with **Holly**, **Vine** and

Cherry Plum) to deal with these states, giving inner peace and freedom from restless pressure and agitation. It helps us to learn to be patient, to be more relaxed and easy-going in outlook. Where someone is slow or less able than we are, instead of blowing up at them Impatiens helps make us able to share our knowledge with them and be helpful to them. Impatiens would make better teachers of us all.

HEATHER *Calluna vulgaris*

The negative Heather state is marked by a great self-preoccupation with a tendency to great talkativeness. Anyone who has ever found themselves held prisoner by a relentless talker who will happily hold their 'victim' rooted to the spot all day long without allowing them to get a word in, has come into contact with a Heather type of person! Deep down, people in this state are lonely, and the loneliness stems from their inability to connect properly with people. They are too self-centred, completely absorbed in their own problems, and feeling a strong need to share these problems with others in order to gain attention. The listener may be initially interested in these problems but soon their smile begins to freeze, their eyes begin to glaze, and they wish they could get away. Should the listener try to talk about themselves or their own problems, the Heather type does not hear, or does not connect; their mind cannot receive incoming calls. It is in many cases the only way a lonely, scared and insecure person can come to feel supported and understood, but forcing themselves on someone in this way often drives that someone away in the process. In extreme cases their drive to seek attention takes the form of feigning sickness, and this hypochondriac tendency may be either conscious or unconscious. Here there is sometimes a fine line between the Heather state and the **Chicory** state, of which more later.

Sometimes animals too can be in need of this remedy, as was the case with Prince, a grey Welsh cob gelding. Fifteen years old and a chronic laminitic, his grass intake was controlled by his owners by sometimes putting him in a bare 'starvation' paddock. Every time the owners passed by, Prince would whinny at them repeatedly to gain their attention. This tendency grew until it got to the stage where they only had to emerge from their back door and he would start calling them from a distance, and once started he would go on for hours. All the juicy haynets, all the toys in the world would not stop him; even when the owners got him a donkey as a companion, he was still the same. On one occasion when the owners had gone out, Prince called to their gardener non-stop for three hours and almost drove the poor woman insane! Prince was prescribed Heather, with the additional change of giving him a close-mesh haynet that would make him take longer to eat his food. After ten days the whinnying had stopped.

5. Oversensitivity to ideas/ influences

People and animals in this group are overly affected by outside stimuli, to which they tend to over-respond in different ways. The remedies in this category are Holly, Walnut, Centaury, and Agrimony.

HOLLY ✷ *Ilex aquifolium*

In the Holly state, the response to outside influences is one of anger, aggressiveness, jealousy and vexation. When we are in this kind of state of mind, any interruptions of our peace, any perceived annoyance or irritation, are met with very strong feelings, which in extreme cases can cause outbursts of physical aggressiveness – from threatening behaviour to abuse to outright violence.

Holly is a very important remedy which should always be kept in stock to deal with those times when we ourselves, or someone around us, becomes very highly susceptible to extreme irritation of this kind. The distress that results from such a state of mind is very considerable, not to mention the possible repercussions of resorting to unruly, aggressive or violent behaviour. Going to prison, losing your job and your home, presents a whole new range of emotional problems that are probably best avoided.

It is often the case that animals come to need Holly. Under certain circumstances – pain, shock, fear, confusion – horses can resort to aggressive behaviour. They do not do so as readily as dogs or cats, being much more flight animals who would rather just run away from any perceived threat. But even a half-power kick from a horse will do a great deal of damage and can even be lethal.

Fighting between horses should not automatically be regarded as Holly behaviour, as they are herd animals with a strong need for social structure, and a pecking-order must often be established by means of physical intimidation. As always with the Bach remedies, it is only when normal emotions and behaviour get out of hand that we can consider we have the 'green light' to go ahead and treat. Sometimes jealousies are sparked off when owners show preferential treatment to a 'favourite' horse, without paying homage to the pecking order, for instance feeding the 'pet' before the other(s) and unwittingly offending the horse(s) higher up the chain of command. Vexation and rage, sometimes with physical violence, can result. In such cases, the practicality and simplicity of the remedies is once again demonstrated, as there is no need to come into actual contact with the aggressive horse.

WALNUT ✸ *Juglans regia*

Here, oversensitivity is expressed in the tendency to be overly swayed or impressed by the various influences acting on us. At times of difficult transition, such as moving to a new home or a new country, getting over changes in life such as divorce, entering life phases such as puberty or the menopause, or generally having to adjust to new and strange circumstances, one may very well experience feelings of vulnerability and diminished self-confidence. It is a state, in short, where we have not yet found our feet.

The most obvious application with horses is in situations where a horse is being introduced to a new home, when it is likely to feel rather overwhelmed by the sudden change in its environment. New horses sometimes appear slightly fretful or withdrawn, perhaps not interested in eating. The remedy would help protect their vulnerable emotional state from unnerving influences, until they have got used to the new place and can feel secure.

CENTAURY ✸ *Centaurium umbellatum*

People whose character tends to the Centaury type are those who are so desperately eager to please those around them that they end up being enslaved by them. In essence, the Centaury nature is truly a virtuous one, and Centauries (nearly always female, incidentally) are generally terribly nice people, very sweet and with a heart of gold, who wish only to make others happy. There should not be anything wrong with being like this! However, such people are all too often dominated by others, often of stronger personality or who manage to be persuasive; these characters may come to take the goodwill of the Centaury type for granted and use them. The Centaury finds it next to impossible to say 'No' to anyone, or to stand up for their own rights; instead they put up with a situation, perhaps accepting it with a sigh, or rationalising it in some way, while getting gradually worn down and losing their vital energy. Eventually life becomes a drudgery, utterly joyless.

In our dealings with animals, the result of a human Centaury state is fairly predictable. Animals will get their own way every time. Horses will quickly learn that a gentle shove with their head can be a means of getting a snack or treat. Of course, the Centaury cannot refuse them, and the behaviour is repeated until the horse is effectively trained to nip or bite when its desires are not immediately met. So many horses are spoiled in this way and become very pushy, and at the root of it all is this basic fault in our attitude. The remedy can be used to adjust the owner's behaviour towards the animal, which, though kindly and sweet, is actually creating real problems for themselves and anyone else who might have to deal with the horse, such as future owners.

AGRIMONY *Agrimonia eupatoria*

The negative Agrimony state is often hard to spot in people, for the simple reason that nobody knows it exists except the person suffering it. The Agrimony type of person is the one who is always cheerful, always seems relaxed, and smiles and jokes a good deal; yet inside themselves, concealed from the eyes of the world, is a painful, gnawing burden of emotional strain. In fact these people are actually very sensitive to outside influences and will often tend to overreact to them, but the reaction is kept underground rather than allowed to surface. This is very harmful to the spirit, and the Agrimony person has to work ever harder to keep up that façade of cheerfulness as the suppressed, denied emotions fester within. They often resort to alcohol and drugs as a means of hiding that inner suffering from the conscious mind, and in fact Agrimony is the first-line remedy for treating inclinations towards addictive habits of this kind. The mind needs to be set free from inner disquiet, and Agrimony allows the troubling feelings to be brought to the surface, where they are made conscious before being released.

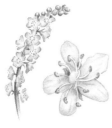

No matter how cheerful and smiling the Agrimony person might appear to other people, if they are harbouring great inner tension they may very easily pass negative body-language and vibrations to their horse and so will never be able to achieve proper relaxation and a real bond with the animal. The Agrimony person cannot 'let go', cannot open up their spirit; there is always that tense little knot inside that prevents them from really participating with all their heart and soul. When the knot is unravelled and the unwanted emotional content is released to the surface of the consciousness, there may be a brief phase of coming to terms with upsetting ideas and feelings; this should not be regarded as a negative state but rather as a positive enlightenment, a cleansing of negativity. A similar effect may take place when taking the remedy **Star of Bethlehem**, which also allows a person to let go of unconscious emotions, sometimes with a great flood of tears, which is then followed by a wonderful sense of tranquillity, as though a huge weight had been taken off the mind.

6. Despondency and despair

In this group are the states of greatest unhappiness, where emotional problems weigh so heavily that they seem impossible to overcome. The remedies in the group are Crab Apple, Oak, Star of Bethlehem, Willow, Sweet Chestnut, Elm, Pine, and Larch.

CRAB APPLE ☆ *Malus sylvestris*

On the psychological level, Crab Apple is the remedy used in cases of self-disgust, where people feel tainted or sullied, or where they feel that there is something in them that is dirty and impure. At one end of the scale, it would be indicated for a person who feels a sense of shame due to a skin condition such as acne; at the other extreme, many women who have been raped or sexually abused would benefit from the remedy's ability to help clean away their sense of having been defiled and dirtied. Either way, Crab Apple is known as a great cleanser.

One of the remarkable things about Crab Apple is its cleansing properties in the physical realm. Added in diluted form to a dressing, it can help draw impurities from a wound; it has also been used to help counter the side-effects of powerful medical drugs, and to ward off impending colds and chills.

Someone emerging from a long period of nursing a very sick animal, having witnessed much pain, suffering and distress, may also benefit from using the remedy to help remove the impression of unpleasantness.

OAK *Quercus robur*

Rather like the Centaury state mentioned earlier, the Oak state is in many ways a virtuous one. An Oak type of person makes a very valuable friend. They display heroic willpower and selfless determination in the face of hardship, and are extremely dependable. But like all good things, this otherwise very laudable state can go wrong. These people will literally work their fingers to the bone for you – and herein lies the flaw in their attitude. The Oak type of person will actually do themselves much damage, both emotionally and, as the years go by, also physically, in the pursuit of their duties. Ultimately they may suffer a terrible decline into depression and despair as their reserves of strength dwindle away.

Oak people are not necessarily ambitious by nature; their motivation is more towards duty to others than to themselves or for their own furtherance. Working as part of a team, they really will give their all. An example of Oak-type problems in riding would be the competition team member who selflessly goes for glory, come what may, and is so intent on doing well for the team that he or she is capable of driving the horse into the ground. Here, the heroic will of the Oak type backfires. In equestrian sport we are not just responsible for ourselves – we are also responsible for the horse. The hard-driving Oak temperament would need to be mellowed slightly to make room for this concept, allowing them to keep up their dedication but with a healthier degree of fun and sportsmanship. The remedy **Vervain** could also be of use here.

STAR OF BETHLEHEM ☆
Ornithogalum umbellatum

Star of Bethlehem, with its wonderful name, is one of the most important of all the Bach flower remedies. It is the remedy for utter sadness, and for the effects of trauma in our lives. It has the ability to reach into deeply buried parts of the unconscious that nothing else can penetrate, healing the direst, grimmest states of despair. It brings true, sometimes quite spectacular release of pent-up emotions. As a retroactive therapy to heal the after-effects of trauma in our lives, no matter how far back, it is extremely effective. All serious traumas leave an imprint on our psyche that remains in place throughout our lives; they cannot be digested, but accumulate in the system and poison us in the same way as toxic elements such as lead. Star of Bethlehem washes away that imprint, bringing immense relief to all who have suffered. As the release happens there may be dreams or conscious memories of the traumatic event. But as always in Bach therapy, it is a very gentle and cathartic process.

For bereavement situations, near-death experiences or serious illness, bad frights, accidents, memories of childhood suffering, e.g. abuse, bullying, terrifying events, it is very much recommended. It is also of great importance in treating emotional states in horses. Any negative state that is in some way rooted in the past, whether it be an instance of cruelty or abuse at the hands of a former owner, a serious injury or shock, or the loss of a beloved companion, is very open to the amazing curative powers of this remedy. Many of the case studies later in this book show the effects of Star of Bethlehem.

WILLOW ✫ *Salix vitellina*

Willow treats the state of despair and despondency that can come on as a result of feeling mistreated either by fate or by specific people or situations. It is a state of smouldering resentment that can drag on and on and from which there seems to be no escape. The result can be great despondency; it can equally be great bitterness and the tendency to attach blame to others for our unlucky fate. Either way it is a very damaging emotional burden.

Some horses have been seen to suffer a Willow state. One of our own ponies, Draco, was an extremely proud character and particularly prone to great resentment and grudge-bearing when he felt cheated or deprived. His case is included in Chapter 6.

SWEET CHESTNUT *Castanea sativa*

Sweet Chestnut deals with a darkened, morbid mood of despair. In this state, we are gripped by black and nihilistic thoughts and a strong sense of faithlessness and aimlessness. Destructive thoughts, of an existential nature rather than the dangerous impulses of **Cherry Plum,** emerge from the blackest parts of the mind and haunt us. Severely painful experiences, such as the death of a loved one, or awful disease-states when the agony is so great as to bring us to question the point of continued existence, or any extreme kind of existential crisis, may give rise to a Sweet Chestnut state. The feeling is one of 'I can't bear this any more; I'm going to break.' The remedy helps us find new reserves of endurance and hope.

Horses can also suffer great hardship, such as when bereaved, that may dictate the use of Sweet Chestnut, helping them to get through the darkest times of their lives.

ELM/PINE
Ulmus procera/Pinus sylvestris

I have grouped these two remedies together as further examples of negative states that can hamper a person's ability to enjoy activities such as riding when they have emotional problems coming at them from other corners of their lives. Elm deals with states of overwhelming responsibility that loom over us and threaten to reduce us to despair, scattering our mental focus and taking the wind out of our sails; Pine treats feelings of guilt, whether justified or not, that have taken root and are undermining our general peace of mind. Either state may create real nervous tension, an unconscious stiffening of the muscles, and a deep inability to relax, conditions that are anathema to riding. So we see that even those states of mind that are not directly related to the field of horses and riders, may still come into play. As I said in the introduction to this book: a happy person makes a happy rider!

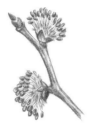

LARCH ✩ *Larix decidua*

This remedy is concerned with states of low self-confidence that are so deep and overwhelming as to bring despair. People suffering this state may often develop self-limiting tendencies. They are loath to participate in activities, or to try anything new, being convinced in advance that they would fail at it. In this it differs from the **Gentian** state; where Gentian merely doubts their abilities, Larch is quite sure that they have none at all. People in the Larch state will often compare themselves unfavourably to others, very quick to find some way in which they would feel or seem inferior. If left to persist, this kind of insecurity will sap the reserves of energy and motivation and lead into what may resemble a **Mustard** state: lethargy, depression and listlessness.

Someone wishing to start, or resume, riding but who feels unable to galvanise themselves into action due to an overpowering sense of inadequacy, or who feels sure that they would be no good at it, would benefit from using this remedy. The Larch type will say things like 'It's just not for me; I simply couldn't do that; I really haven't got what it takes to get on the back of a horse.' Equally, someone who is already riding but feels hampered by a sense of low self-confidence and is convinced they can progress no further, would find in Larch the boost they need to overcome that mental block.

7. Overconcern for others' welfare

We should be careful not to let the title of this final group of remedies mislead us. We have already seen how the remedy **Red Chestnut** is indicated for fears relating to the safety or welfare of a loved one. Surely, then, that remedy should have been included in this group rather than put into the group FEAR? Dr Bach was a particular kind of thinker, and sometimes we have to stop and consider his meaning – in this instance, what he meant by overconcern for others' welfare. We must remember that the good doctor spent much of his life analysing, subdividing and classifying emotional states, and that his definitions and headings can be very subtle. What he categorised under the above heading was a collection of five mental/emotional states whereby people tend to dominate others; they interfere in others' affairs out of a belief that they know best. They can be completely thoughtless, overpowering and even dictatorial, failing to consider and respect other people's individual wishes and needs. To simplify its definition, we might wish to re-classify this group as 'over-involvement with others' affairs'.

The five remedies in this group are Beech, Rock Water, Vervain, Vine, and Chicory.

BEECH *Fagus sylvatica*

The Beech remedy helps those who are overly critical and intolerant of others, ever seeking to bend and shape others' will. They have a very negative outlook and constantly find fault with everything around them. It is a somewhat arrogant and judgemental state of mind. Dissatisfaction, negativity, brittleness and closed-mindedness are the hallmarks of the Beech person. The remedy works well with others such as **Agrimony** and **Star of Bethlehem** to release the hidden inner sadness and past experiences that may have contributed to the development of such a state.

Animals in need of Beech will display signs of intolerance towards people or other animals. Where a dog might growl aggressively at the sight of someone it dislikes or is suspicious of, such as the hated vet, a horse is more likely to respond in fear.

Where this remedy is most useful in horse treatment is for cases of intolerance between horses themselves, for instance where pecking order gets out of hand – here remedies such as **Holly** and **Vine** are also useful (see Chapter 3).

ROCK WATER

Unique among the Bach remedies, Rock Water does not actually come from a plant. Instead it is derived from natural spring water sources traditionally believed to carry healing powers. For many centuries people have believed in the curative properties of certain water sources; the most outstanding example being the legendary waters of Lourdes in France. Then there is the historic tradition of bathing in, or drinking, the water of spas, to which was attributed the relief of many chronic disease states.

This remedy is used to treat people who are too hard on themselves, who go out of their way to choose an ascetic, self-punitive and spartan way of life. Frequently, the true motivation of such people is their buried desire to inspire others by their example, and they secretly hope and demand that the rest of society should do as they do, think as they think. And therein lies the element of overconcern for others' welfare. The keywords to understanding this remedy-state are rigidity, discipline, extreme self-control. People who fanatically adhere to restrictive diets, hard exercise regimes, cold showers, puritanical sexual abstinence, and so on, could (at the point where they recognise they have a problem) benefit from Rock Water. The remedy serves to take the edge off their rather harsh view of life.

In the treatment of animals, there is relatively little indication for this remedy. A possible example would, however, be the trotting-horse. Horses that are bred and trained to compete in trotting racing events are so highly disciplined that when they retire, their new owners may experience great difficulty in getting them to move at a slow trot, canter or gallop. All they can do is what they have been trained for. Rock Water might well be indicated to smooth away the impact of that rigorous training, allowing the horse access to easier paces that should come completely naturally to it but have been suppressed by endlessly repeated habit.

VERVAIN ✫ *Verbena officinalis*

This is the remedy for over-enthusiasm. Vervain treats states of mind that render us overly energised, 'hyped up', hyperactive. Very manic people, or manic-depressives in their manic phase, can benefit from the remedy. The Vervain state is often seen in comedy, with actors such as Jerry Lewis, Robin Williams, Eddie Murphy and Jim Carrey exploiting their wildly over-the-top roles to the full. While the fictitious characters these actors portray in their films are amusing, in real life, people who behave in this way can run into problems. In day-to-day living such individuals consume huge amounts of energy and may hit the depths when their resources run low, leading to nervous tension, depression and sometimes even a breakdown. The remedy Vervain will help to calm the tendency to hyperactive behaviour, ensuring that energy reserves will be more cautiously utilised.

Horses, especially young horses that are absolutely bursting with energy, may need calming occasionally when their energy levels border on the excessive. In jumping, an over-enthusiastic horse may be so eager that it takes a jump too soon. After an event, a horse may be very worked up and still wanting to go. Or it might be that your horse constantly wants to break into a fast pace when all you want is a gentle hack. Any forms of over-enthusiastic behaviour, very common in horses, may be treated with Vervain. Of course responsible owners should always be sure that the energy content of the feed they are giving the horse is not excessive for the amount of work he is expected to do, as hyperactivity problems can and sometimes do arise from inappropriate nutrition.

VINE ✫ *Vitis vinifera*

When people show signs of dominant, ruthless or tyrannical behaviour, Vine is the indicated remedy. People in the Vine state will tend to seize control of situations and also people, imposing their will even when not desired by others. If we look, we can see the state taking hold of people at every level of life to varying degrees: some teachers, police officers, parents, husbands/wives, officials, can be highly intractable, petty-minded people who use whatever power they have to dominate those around them. It can grow to a very extreme state, Adolf Hitler being one of the more prominent Vine types of recent times. The entire history of mankind is peppered with famous names who were power-hungry, overbearing, and violently abusive – all Vine types. Abuses of human rights, and the actions of 'control-freaks', are Vine characteristics. People who abuse children and animals are displaying the same dreadful urges.

Of course, we humans are far more cruel, far more violent and potentially evil than are any other creatures on earth. Nonetheless, it can happen that animals, too, fall into negative states of mind that involve abusive and controlling behaviour and may be treated with the Vine remedy. We have observed horses pushing the boundaries of their herd leadership far beyond what was necessary to maintain order, actually preventing other horses from reaching their food just for the sake of it. In other cases the Vine state can be seen working hand-in-hand with jealousy, for instance the horse that will not allow another to approach the owner at the fence. Here Vine and **Holly** would work well together. Occasionally, if a horse has been allowed to impose himself too much on the owner/rider, the latter not commanding enough respect, aggressive and domineering behaviour may emerge. This kind of state really cannot be allowed to continue. Retraining can help, but the situation will return if the owner does not address his or her own attitude. It may be that they are lacking in confidence, or unable to impose their personality to any effect. Of course, here again the Bach remedies are most useful in dealing with these negative situations.

CHICORY *Cichorium intybus*

Chicory is for those who try to bind others to them in a possessive way. They share with all of us the normal need for affection and love, but they combine it with the need to control and influence. A Chicory type has to be the centre of attention, and though they are willing to give, if they do not get the required response in return they may become very resentful and self-pitying. Emotional blackmail and feigning of illness to gain attention are among the extremes of behaviour to which the Chicory type may resort.

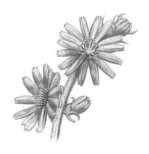

The remedy works well in conjunction with **Willow**, for resentment, and also with **Heather**. Chicory could be seen as an extension of certain aspects of the Heather state. It rests on the same desire for attention; but by the time the state of mind has dwindled into the Chicory state, there is a greater urgency, a more pressing need to get and keep that attention by whatever means necessary. The state also shows a **Holly** side in its tendency toward jealousy: animals who become resentful, moody and perhaps refuse to eat because the owner showed greater affection to another in the pack or herd, are displaying combined signs of Chicory, Holly and Willow.

RESCUE REMEDY☆

Rescue Remedy is perhaps the most famous of all the Bach flower remedies. It is often the remedy that introduces people to the Bach system. It is not truly a thirty-ninth remedy, but a composite of **Rock Rose** for panic, **Cherry Plum** for loss of self-control, **Impatiens** for great tension, **Clematis** for faintness and withdrawal, and **Star of Bethlehem** for shock and trauma. It is very useful in emergencies and can be administered for just about any dramatic or frightening situation. It has been argued that using the same five remedies for all such situations is failing to take the individual patient into account, and that Rescue Remedy is tantamount to shooting with a shotgun, random and inaccurate. To this I would respond that a shotgun may not be a rifle but is nonetheless a highly effective tool in an emergency! Between them, these five remedies have most of such situations covered, even if, say, only two of the five remedies are actually doing the work. The goal in a crisis is to get the patient calm and safe as quickly as possible, and the powerful package that is Rescue Remedy is the perfect formula to achieve that at extremely short notice. The remedy can actually save lives when given at the right moment. It also can be used in the aftermath of a trauma, say, for a person or animal who is in deep shock, and then for the days and weeks that follow. In immediate crisis situations dosage can be generous: four drops every ten to thirty minutes until results are obtained.

For riders, a slim 10ml bottle of Rescue Remedy can be carried in the smallest pocket. For extra protection from broken glass in the event of a fall, the bottle could be wrapped in cloth or bubble-wrap, if so desired. Alternatively it can be stored in a saddlebag or pouch, where it could live permanently. I would recommend that anyone venturing out on horseback, whether alone or in a group, even for a short hack, should be suitably 'armed' with a bottle of Rescue Remedy.

RESCUE CREAM ✯

This very popular addition to the Bach remedy collection is a soothing all-purpose cream containing the five regular constituents of **Rescue Remedy**, with the addition of **Crab Apple** for its cleansing properties. The cream can be applied topically to all skin conditions such as minor cuts, grazes, burns, cold-burns, blisters, dried or chapped skin, and rashes. The non-animal-fat cream base contains honey, which on its own is recognised as a good healer for skin abrasions and the like.

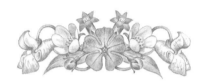

CHAPTER THREE

THE HORSE

Once we have gained a good knowledge of the Bach flower remedies, with the emphasis on the most useful ones for the horse-rider duo, we are in theory ready to start using them. Mindful of the various problems we have been experiencing with our horse, and full of the best intentions, we put a collection of remedy bottles into our bag and march off down to the stable-yard, where our horse awaits. We stare at the horse; the horse turns to stare at us. It is remedy time!

Or is it? Have we really thought about the nature of whatever 'problem' it is that we are experiencing? Do we really understand what is going on? What is the underlying psychology? Are we really, truly, honestly, objective about our own attitude to the horse? Do we really, truly, objectively know the mind and character of the horse? Do we fully understand its reactions?

If any of these matters raises a doubt in our mind, we need to put the remedies away for a minute and reflect. Take a step or two back from the horse. What is this animal that stands before us, so familiar and yet so strange? How did it evolve to be the way it is? How does it differ from horses in the wild? In what ways does it resemble, and in what ways does it differ from, us humans? How does it regard me, its keeper?

Many people make mistakes when it comes to interpreting their animal's way of thinking and subsequent behaviour. One trap we often fall into is to travel the well-worn anthropomorphic route, which is to assume that if an animal such as a horse has emotions and feelings, these must be the same as our own human emotions and feelings. This view completely fails to take into account any of the biological and/or evolutionary differences between what are in fact two very different species. The other trap is to look at the animal from a strictly behavioural, cause-and-effect angle such as that propounded by a certain well-known American psychologist, which basically reduces animals to the level of inanimate robots and fails to take into account or even acknowledge the subtle inner workings of the animal's mind, such as its capacity to remember, to be happy or to be sad. This attitude to animals, hardly surprisingly, forms a rigid rational justification in the minds of many for the horrible, shameful treatment that animals often have to suffer at the hands of humans.

Neither of these opposite viewpoints will do; a line has to be drawn down the middle that allows us to understand the animal – in this instance the horse – first as a horse and not as a human, but also as a deeply sensitive and emotionally aware creature that responds to love, has real needs and is capable of suffering emotional imbalances just as we are.

To get into the mind of animals, sometimes it may serve to look at a certain species in the context of another. Look at dogs, for instance. Dogs and humans have a great many mental/emotional characteristics in common, and the two species are probably more closely matched in this respect than are horses and humans. For a start, the modern dog tends to live in the house with us and share more hours of the day with us than most of our horses do, picking up on a lot of our traits and mannerisms. But more importantly, humans and canines share in being predatory pack animals, omnivorous animals with similarities in dentition and digestive system. Like us, dogs tend to be more combative, more prone to violence as a means of self-defence, than horses. In the wild, our ancestors and our dogs' ancestors would have been out after the same prey. And amongst that prey would have been the ancestors of our horses.

So our horse is actually fundamentally quite a different order of animal from us. As a herbivorous prey animal the equine species evolved, from the tiny, toed *Eohippus* of prehistoric times to the modern *Equus caballus*, to live on its wits and be constantly on the watch for predators, ever ready to flee at the first sign of trouble. The horse's social structure evolved so as to protect the herd, prospective leaders competing against each other to establish a natural pecking-order and the most defensive young stallions forming a vanguard against predators. A horse left on its own, without the protective circle of the herd around it, had little chance of survival. Many thousands of years of formation have thus shaped the horse into a very social animal that derives comfort from the company of the herd and will bond strongly with other horses, yet is also a nervy animal whose primary instinct in the face of a perceived threat is to escape, to put as much distance between the herd and the 'predator' as possible.

From this simple portrait of the horse we can see its principal characteristics, which have remained unchanged since prehistory:
- the herd instinct to stick together and follow one another;
- the desire for security in numbers, the emergence of leaders to hold the herd together;
- the liking for comforting group routine; and
- the extremely highly developed sense of danger – the 'switch' that turns them from lazy grazers with not a care in the world to startled, wide-eyed, rapidly disappearing specks on the horizon at the drop of a hat!

As a 'flight' rather than a 'fight' animal, the horse's threshold of pain is considerably lower than, say, that of a German Shepherd dog. And as we can see from the tiny inputs from leg and hand that are required to control the horse in riding, this is an animal that is very highly sensitive to touch in general. Lay a hand on the back of a horse that is even slightly nervous and notice the big twitch in the muscles. Even a fly landing on the horse's skin can have this effect.

This sensitivity is more than matched by the sensitivity of the horse's emotions. The horse's mentality is a very complex and delicate one indeed. It is all too easy to 'bruise' them emotionally, and with their long memories they can be badly damaged and scarred. Dealing with horses is a difficult business, in which we must walk something of a tightrope to do things correctly. On the one hand we have to handle them with kid gloves lest we traumatise them. Punishing undesirable behaviour will in many cases serve only to exacerbate a problem by compounding the underlying fearful emotions. We have to be extremely calm, patient and understanding. But on the other hand, as part of the relationship we have struck up with them, we are perceived by them as part of their herd; and as such we must gain the respect of these much bigger, stronger animals in order to be in control of them and preserve our own health and safety!

There are many pitfalls, and many issues to deal with in our partnership with horses. If we break them down to specific situations in our everyday life with horses we can isolate particular problems so as to consider them in the light of the Bach flower remedies.

Your new horse

We can start experiencing problems right from the very start, before we even so much as have a horse fitted for a saddle! Consider the 'new horse' scenario. When you pull into the yard, drop the tailgate on the trailer and your new acquisition steps rather nervously out into the environment that is to be his home, in most cases there will be a good deal of apprehension in the mind of the horse. The first thing to do is make the horse feel comfortable so that he can get on with the business of settling in. You will have his stable ready for him and a little bit to eat, so that rather than let him straight out with other horses, he can be brought in and allowed to understand that here is a nice, comforting and protective environment in which to feel secure. The settling-in process may take as little as three days or as long as three months, depending entirely on the individual nature of the horse. To lessen the impact of all the bewildering new sights, smells, sounds and the sense of sudden change, it could be a good idea to give the horse four or five drops of the Bach remedy **Walnut**, four times a day in his water or on a chunk of carrot throughout the settling-in period. If he exhibits signs of nervousness and agitation, **Mimulus**, or for more panicky states of real fear, **Rock Rose**, will soothe and calm. I personally think that a little dose of **Star of Bethlehem** is a good way to introduce any horse into a new environment, giving an immediate positive sense and warding off any feelings of trauma from the big change in its life.

Pretty soon, if there are other horses around, the new arrival needs to make their acquaintance. The others will be highly curious about him and will also want to get the pecking-order situation clear from the start. This is all quite normal; they need to get themselves sorted out and generally it is little of our business. However, you want the new horse to get the best start in his new home. If it seems he is excessively frightened or dominated by the 'old hands', a fear remedy like **Mimulus**, or even just the general **Rescue Remedy**, will do wonders for his confidence and overall first impressions of the place.

As time passes and your new horse begins to realise that this new place is obviously going to be his permanent home, he may feel a sense of separation from his former home and companions. This is especially true of horses who are a bit older and have perhaps spent years under their previous ownership, where they may have formed bonds with other horses, or people, or where their general environment made them feel safe and protected. **Honeysuckle** is the remedy for this kind of homesick, nostalgic state. In some cases they really may pine, and some owners are made to feel rather guilty for taking them away from their old, happy home. **Sweet Chestnut**, **Star of Bethlehem**, and **Gorse** are all useful for dealing with this sort of horsey depression. If all the other conditions are right, before too long the horse will adapt quite happily to his new situation and be able to settle in and make friends with everyone around, horse and human.

Sweet Chestnut

Boxing and transportation

Although most horses are quite used to getting in and out of trailers and stables, it is against their nature to walk straight into a narrow space, through a doorway, or into a dark room, without a real sense of trepidation. After all, there could be a lion or a wolf in there! These are both highly unnatural situations for the horse, whose instinct tells him that these places, far from the protective shelters that you see them as, are bad and suspicious. When being introduced to a new stable, or being trailered for the first time, many horses will freak out completely and resist even the most juicy titbits intended to lure them in. Putting a rope behind the horse's rump and forcing him in may do the trick, but the most humane and gentle way is surely to address the emotion at the bottom of the problem: namely his quite understandable fear.

As is so often the case with horses, the remedies to consider are **Rock Rose** for more short-term acute states of panic, where you need to get him in quite quickly and wish for rapid results, and **Mimulus** to deal with a chronic, ongoing repetition of the problem. The two remedies could be given together if desired. Once the horse has understood that there is nothing to fear, and carrots await him inside, the problem is solved without the need for brute force or loss of temper. Quelling his fearful state also helps guard against potentially self-damaging attacks of panic whilst on the move inside the trailer. We have seen a solid aluminium trailer with its ceiling punched through as though by a cannon shell after a horse panicked inside. If you think your horse is capable of violent loss of self-control, **Cherry Plum** would be an excellent remedy to give before (perhaps starting a few days in advance) and during transportation.

Shoeing

Visits from the farrier are not always welcome as far as horses are concerned, and many owners dread shoeing-time, knowing that their horses are going to misbehave. In some cases, their behaviour makes it impossible to do the work.

Again, this situation, and the need for iron shoes, is something that we impose upon the horse as part of his unnatural role working for us. It is, however, something we do for the horse's own good. But naturally horses don't see it that way! It is their instinct to be afraid of the farrier, as it is their instinct to fear any intrusion into their lives. In most cases, training and experience make the horse realise that nothing is wrong, there is no real threat, and the easiest option is to comply. But there will always be those horses who rebel, making the experience a difficult one for all concerned, making themselves suffer unnecessary emotional trauma. It is a vicious circle – the more the horse fights back, the more impossible the job becomes, and the more the horse remembers this is the way to prevent us from doing this awful thing to him. It may only take two or three failed attempts to 'train' a horse into being utterly, permanently impossible to shoe without having him powerfully sedated by a vet.

Enter the Bach flowers. To pick the right remedy we must ask, what is the underlying source of the struggle? In addition to the standard fear remedies of **Rock Rose** and **Mimulus** we might have to consider others. To get the message across to young, impulsive horses that shoeing is not a thing to be dreaded, **Chestnut Bud** is a useful remedy that helps prevent repetition of the error and encourages training to sink in. Did the farrier ever hurt the horse, either intentionally, which he might have felt was the best way to gain its respect, or unintentionally? Perhaps the horse is full of resentment towards him: **Willow** and **Holly** may very well serve here, lessening the horse's feelings of hostility. Alternatively, you may have to speak to previous owners to find out whether the horse may have had a particular trauma that he associates with being manhandled by a stranger. If this is so, horses can carry this memory with them always, and warning lights will come on in the horse's mind at the merest approach from the farrier and for that matter the horse dentist, the vet and anyone else he decides to mistrust. You would do well to add **Star of Bethlehem** to your list of remedies here.

The above solutions apply equally to problems with tying-up. If a horse has been left tied to a wall for a long time, or this has been part of past maltreatment, he may associate it with pain and fear. Or it may just be a case of intolerance and indignation at being restricted (read humiliated) like this – **Holly/Beech**.

Beech

Training and handling

When it comes to general handling and trying to make the horse do as we wish, we can come across many obstacles. Before we can even make a start, we have to catch the horse – and for many owners even this most basic thing is a problem. A horse that will not be caught usually has, in its way of thinking, a valid reason for acting this way.

Does the horse normally let himself be caught? If so and this is unusual behaviour, he could actually be suffering from some physical disorder and in pain and, knowing that your act of grooming him or riding him is going to be unpleasant, he understandably wishes to avoid this. It would not be a bad idea to call the vet in cases where a horse persists in not being caught (assuming you and the vet and a couple of assistants can corner the animal so that he can be inspected!). Once given the all-clear from the vet, you can consider other reasons for the problem.

Has the horse developed some fear of the rope or headcollar? **Rock Rose/Mimulus**. Is this a new horse? Perhaps he has been terrorised by people trying to catch him in the past – **Star of Bethlehem**. Consider also that you are being used! Blackmail is not unknown in horses, to say the least, and perhaps there is something of a manipulative **Chicory** dynamic at work, the horse enjoying being the centre of attention and willing to sell himself to you only at the price of a double handful of chopped carrots. Do not underestimate their ability to be devious!

Horses are often hard to lead properly, perhaps going off in different directions when they see tempting bits of grass; perhaps barging across you and threatening to crush your toes. This is a real nuisance, potentially dangerous and needs to be dealt with. It is not based upon fear – quite the opposite. The horse has not fully absorbed the lessons of training. So think: is the horse always eager, always 'hyper', always rushing ahead? If so, consider the remedy **Vervain** for over-enthusiasm. If it were not for the fact that eagerness is a most desirable trait for racehorses, this would be the solution to the problem of leading them, which often necessitates three or four people hanging on for all they are worth! Is the horse being youthfully exuberant, impulsive, perhaps seeming clumsy and rather dull-witted? **Chestnut Bud** would help him to better absorb the lessons of training and experience.

Think carefully and be objective in regard to the next question. Is the horse just playing you up and imposing himself on you? Perhaps he needs **Vine**, as he sees himself as your leader, rather than the other way round. Most likely in this scenario, however, it is you, the handler, that needs a boost of self-confidence and authoritativeness, without which the horse may not ever respect you!

This is a vital point. It applies in all cases of aggression, for instance aggression around food in the stable, or with horses that are prone to bite, and is of the utmost importance. We should remember that, as an honorary member of the herd, we need to maintain our own position within it. Horses will kick, nip and bite each other in their competitions for superiority within the herd, and to hold on to their top roles once they have won them. A horse that treats us with such contempt is trying to take us down a notch in the hierarchy, or reminding us of our lowly position, at which point it is up to us to ensure that we rise quickly back to the top of the herd! We should be the leaders, and that is quite final. Sometimes we spoil horses with treats, thinking the horse will love us for it, and in so doing, giving on demand, we unwittingly lower ourselves in the horse's estimation. We therefore need to think about ourselves, think about our own command of the horse's respect. Are we lacking in the necessary self-confidence and strength of will and personality to win the respect of such a big animal? See the next chapter.

Riding

Problems in riding can generally be broken down into napping, spooking, rearing, bucking, and bolting. They can be attributed to the horse's instinctive fear-driven urge to run away from trouble, a lack of training, a combination of the above or other factors. Dealing with these other factors first, unpredictable or extreme behaviour could be caused by physical problems: e.g. pain in the mouth made worse by the movement of the bit, or back pain. It has been suggested that the 'cold-backed' horse who dislikes the saddle may be suffering from rheumatism. As always, it is advisable to have the horse checked over by a vet to ensure that there is no physical problem underlying the riding troubles.

Once we have the green light to consider the problem as a mental/emotional one, we can start thinking about our choice of remedies. In most cases we will be thinking in terms of fear. A horse that is very nervous and easily startled by the slightest thing may suddenly veer sideways, bolt, whirl around or even rear up. When one considers that much of our leisure riding in Britain involves negotiating busy roads and motorists who are either unaware of the risks with horses or too impatient and aggressive to care, the chances of serious accident are high. Horses that are highly strung and constantly on edge will respond to **Rock Rose** very well. The remedy helps take the edge off the horse's tendency to panic, keeping it calm, focused and under the control of the rider.

Napping may be born of fear, in which case **Rock Rose** and **Mimulus** will prove very useful. For instance, when the horse is being ridden out from the security of the stable-yard, it may suddenly stop, refuse to go on, or try to turn back because it suddenly feels insecure. Similarly, it may be that a particular landmark, such as a flapping sign, swaying bush or the milk float that is always parked outside number 32 when we ride by at 10.15 every morning, is a great source of terror in the horse's mind! Horses can seemingly spook for no apparent reason, which can be very dangerous and unpredictable. The horse is so tuned to its environment, so watchful for any possible threat, that the tiniest little thing can spell danger: a sweet wrapper stuck in the hedgerow, a small bird flying past, a banging gate, may all trigger a fearful reaction.

Whatever the manifestation, any chronically fearful state can be very successfully treated with whichever fear remedy we think is most applicable to the individual case. Then again, such problems may be a sign of the horse playing the rider up and being silly, or being dominant. The rider may be lacking in confidence, of course, and passing his or her negative vibrations of insecurity and lack of control to the horse, who naturally tries to exploit the situation. A rider who is too vulnerable to

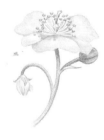

Rock Rose

nervousness is telling the horse: 'I can't handle this situation. You be the leader, I'll just sit here.'

The same applies to bucking. As long as we know our horse is healthy and free from pain, being fed the right food and getting enough exercise, we might consider the possibility that the horse is trying to get rid of the annoying human on his back. **Holly** and **Vine** would be given if it is a case of dominant aggression; **Beech** would be appropriate in cases of disrespectful intolerance; **Vervain** for over-exuberance; and **Chestnut Bud** if the horse is immaturely 'forgetting itself' and too impulsive. Once again, the rider's job is to stay in command of the situation, keep the horse going forward, perhaps pull him round in circles and generally stay on top of things to show the horse who is in charge.

In the next chapter we look at ways to help ourselves, as riders and handlers, to overcome problems with self-confidence.

Accidents and emergencies

By and large, all emergency situations are going to provoke the same general sort of emotional reactions in a horse, namely terror and panic. Whether a fire breaks out in the stable-yard, causing mass pandemonium, or a horse suffers a crippling colic attack, complications in foaling or is hit by a car, for the purposes of the Bach flower remedy user the responses can be treated in the same way. Trying to calm and reassure a sick, injured or otherwise distressed horse whilst waiting for the vet to arrive is much aided by the use of **Rescue Remedy**. Its handy five-in-one format allows for very rapid and efficient administration and takes away the need to sift through a box of thirty-eight bottles, our mind racing as we try to come up with a prescription.

One tip: in emergency situations you may find that the only way to administer the remedy is neat from the bottle into the mouth. Caution should be exercised: a horse that is panic-stricken may bite off and swallow the glass dropper tube when you try to get the remedy into its mouth, which would be disastrous. If in doubt, unscrew the cap and pour the remedy straight from the bottle into the mouth, rubbing it into the tongue and gums as much as you can to get it into the bloodstream quickly. If you are able to insert your fingers into the side of the mouth you can offset the chances of being bitten; but then a little bite is nothing compared to possibly saving the horse's life. Don't worry about being generous with the remedy; if half the bottle is gone by the time the vet arrives, you will not have harmed the horse.

Horses living alone and stress-related habits

An 'only horse', who lives without the company of other horses, is not necessarily bound to be unhappy as is often thought. Horses will adopt any form of company as part of their herd. Some owners without the facilities for two horses even find that keeping a few chickens is a good way of providing some company for the horse. Then, of course, there is the owner and any other humans who are about. However, without sufficient stimulation and companionship, it is quite possible for horses to become lonely, bored and thus develop bad habits such as weaving and crib-biting, or fall into states of withdrawal and depression.

Weaving, crib-biting and other boredom/stress-related habits are notoriously difficult things to cure. For Bach treatment, one would, as always, need to determine the exact cause of the problem, and if the cause is poor management of the horse, then that will have to be sorted out as a first priority. The Bach flower remedies are not to be used as a replacement for proper care! However, sometimes these things persist no matter what.

For the horse who never seems to relax, never seems content, is always itching for something and getting flustered by long periods of inactivity, **Impatiens** and **Vervain** will help reduce the stress it is suffering.

Compulsive, repetitive behaviour such as crib-biting and pacing up and down may be addressed by such remedies as **Scleranthus** where there is constant vacillation from one thing to another. **Cherry Plum** could be given for destructive impulses, and **Star of Bethlehem** and **Mustard** if the horse is very depressed. **Agrimony** may possibly be indicated if it seems that the horse is suffering from vague inner tension.

The tendency to fall into cycles of meaningless behaviour may mark a **Wild Rose** state of severe boredom and withdrawal. The remedy would also benefit horses that just stand and stare disconsolately into space for hours on end – as would **Clematis**. If you think the horse misses company that it used to enjoy and had grown to depend upon,

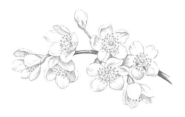

Cherry Plum

Honeysuckle would be of great use to boost the horse's interest in the here and now and bring increased happiness.

Of course, many of these bad habits can also occur when horses are together; sometimes they learn from each other, imitating another horse's crib-biting, for example. This may be even harder to control, but one could think of adding **Chestnut Bud** to the above list, to help deal with the added element of immature, follow-my-leader-orientated, impulsive repetition.

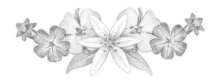

CHAPTER FOUR

THE RIDER/HANDLER

The bond we have forged with horses over the centuries is a complicated one. On one level we are the horse's Lord and Master, and we expect and demand that he comply with our wishes. In this sense our relationship with horses echoes the original, less-than-altruistic motivation for forming such a link with another species. Our ancestors effectively enlisted a wild animal to exploit its strength and its endurance. The horse was an invaluable tool, and played an enormous part in the formation of human civilisation. It helped us to till the earth and learn about agriculture; it made it possible for us to defeat enemies in battle and establish law and order; and by allowing us to cover long distances it permitted the spread of settlements and the establishment of supply and communication routes from place to place. We owe a lot to horses. Try to imagine history without them. The horse also served, as it still sometimes does, as a food source for ourselves and various other animals that we have similarly enlisted for our purposes, notably dogs. So it was in one way all very practical and utilitarian.

On another level, humans experience very strong emotional ties with their horses. Perhaps this tendency has increased as our dependency on the horse as a working tool has decreased over the course of the twentieth century. Many people form lifelong friendships with their horses, are utterly devoted to them and even believe they experience telepathic links with them. When their horses die, people are often severely upset, and behave almost as though they had lost a family member.

This complex, two-way bond between human and horse is very much reflected when we come to consider the use of the Bach flower remedies, or indeed any question of horse/rider psychology. What we are effectively doing is balancing the relationship between the two species. Each side must have trust in, and yet respect for, the other. Any disturbance in that balance can have adverse effects: a fragile state of affairs indeed!

The mental link between horse and rider is such that the rider's emotional state is utterly crucial to the ability to ride well and in such a way as to make it a pleasant and safe experience for both parties concerned. One cannot achieve this mutually comfortable 'link-up' unless all barriers, blockages, in the mind and emotions – fear, worry, imaginings – are overcome. This rather cruel yet unavoidable fact can be a mind-bogglingly overwhelming stumbling-block for any rider or handler who is nervous. The more we try to force ourselves to calm down, the more tense we become, and the more the tension is picked up on by the horse. The horse, depending on its individual character, will then often tend to behave skittishly, fearfully, or stubbornly with us, and this in turn will compound our own sense of fear, doubt and frustration. Catch 22!

In the previous chapter we looked at how the negative emotions and impulses in the horse can be addressed by the Bach flower remedies; now we turn to the other half of the duo, the human.

Getting in the saddle

Nervousness has to be overcome right from the start. In riding, we are not going to go very far unless we can make that first step: to get on the back of a horse! Yet many people who want to start riding, as well as people who already have experience, develop basic fears and worries that prevent them from making progress. For beginners who are just rather nervous, the standard fear remedy **Mimulus** will be of benefit. If fear is much more acute and borders on terror, try **Rock Rose** instead. But the underlying reasons may be more subtle and go to a deeper level of the personality. A general lack of confidence in oneself will certainly come to the fore when starting out in riding, as it does with learner drivers. Here, **Larch** is of great benefit. If we are convinced in advance that we will fail, there is a strong chance that either we will fail as predicted, or that we will not even have the courage and incentive to try. For those who are not so much afraid as unmotivated, **Clematis**, for the daydreamers, or **Wild Oat** for the underachievers who stifle potential talent, will help give the necessary focus and drive.

Larch

The benevolent dictator

As we have seen, horses are very aware of herd hierarchy. It is their nature to assume a certain role in the herd, climbing over those members who are seen to be weak and yielding. That member could be you! A lack of confidence in ourselves means that we are not putting out the signals worthy of a herd leader, and the result will often be misbehaviour in the horse. There is no point treating the horse if we are the ones at fault. **Mimulus** and **Larch** will help enormously here also. **Cerato** is another first-line remedy for this kind of state, helping with self-assertiveness. If we have trouble commanding authority, another excellent remedy is **Centaury**. The same remedy would apply if we tend excessively to let the horse have its own way when it 'asks' for a treat or to go on the grass for a nibble, which gradually erodes our authority.

If setbacks are undermining our confidence and the horse is creating further setbacks by exploiting that lack, the negative spiral can be broken using **Gentian**. Cool, collected confidence is our goal, and it will allow us to exude the manners of a leader, exert the control we need over the horse, and keep our head under stress. Remember that there is nothing wrong with being the horse's boss. The horse wants, needs, and thrives on having a strong leader who will show it which way to go, take the initiative and yet remain calm and gentle.

The road

Riding on the road is probably the most dangerous activity most riders undertake. In Britain and elsewhere, many accidents take place each year involving horses and motorists, often with fatalities. Yet for many of us, going out on the road, even just to get from one bridlepath to another, is inevitable. Even experienced riders who are not normally nervous can feel great trepidation as the country roads they use from day to day become steadily busier, cars get faster and quieter, making them harder to hear approaching, and drivers get more aggressive and less and less in tune with country ways. Balancing our fears and trying to transmit positive vibrations to the horse when we feel in real danger is not always easy.

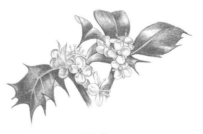

Holly

Rock Rose will serve to take the edge off our fear; **Cherry Plum** will remove the unconscious urge to let panic dictate our actions. These are both contained in the **Rescue Remedy** formula, giving us another good reason to carry it when out riding. Should we become angered by bad drivers and feel like shouting or waving our fist at them, **Holly** will help us keep our calm – not for the benefit of the drivers, but rather for that of the horse and ourselves.

The show-ring

A far less dangerous, though equally nerve-racking environment, is the show scenario. As a rider performing in front of a crowd, we are likely to feel nervous; in fact this nervousness will most likely have been dragging on for days or weeks, depending on our experience. It is a good idea to start taking **Mimulus** several days before the event. **Larch** will help for those who feel embarrassed by being watched, **Gentian** for those whose confidence goes to pieces after losing points or missing a jump. **Impatiens** will help with feelings of irritation against the horse when it does not perform as well as it did in the privacy of the school, and also with the sense of anger that we feel against ourselves for making a mistake or perceiving that we are under-performing.

Sometimes the sheer pressure on the mind can be so overwhelming that the rider's mind becomes hazy. We might need to remember the layout of a course or the sequence in a dressage test, for instance, and suddenly go into a panic when our mind goes blank at a crucial point. For that kind of overwhelming pressure, **Elm** is useful, helping to keep things ordered in the mind and everything in perspective.

If we have experienced these kinds of difficulties in past shows and would like to use the Bach remedies to improve our chances in future shows, we should try to think back and pinpoint the exact nature of the problem: exactly how we felt, when and why. As we were reacting under pressure and those pressures are likely to be replicated more or less exactly from show to show, there is a good chance that we can predict how we will feel in advance. So if we feel we did badly due to, say, nervousness, lack of confidence, falling apart, losing our temper and going blank, **Mimulus**, **Larch**, **Gentian**, **Impatiens** and **Elm** could be taken in combination in advance. If we thought these were quite deep-seated tendencies within our personality, we could start two or three weeks ahead of the dreaded date to make sure we were really on top of the problem. Then all that remains is to treat the horse's neuroses too! And to try to ride well, naturally...

After a fall

Whatever stage of the game we are at, at some point we are probably going to fall off our horse. This is a simple fact of life, to which we should all try to adjust. It is something that happens to everyone somewhere along the line, and although people can be injured in unlucky cases, most spills involve little more than a few bruises, a dented ego and sand in your teeth. More confident riders will generally be able to dust themselves off and get straight back into the saddle, concentrating on the business of sorting out whatever error of judgement caused the fall. Others, however, can respond very badly to these frightening incidents, and be put off riding again – in some cases permanently.

If we have suffered a blow to our confidence after falling off, a key remedy to take is **Gentian** for dealing with setbacks. If the idea of getting back into the saddle causes trembling and panic, **Rock Rose** can be taken several times a day to quell the fear and will also work quickly if we take a bottle with us to the stable yard. Again, our little cure-all **Rescue Remedy** will serve us well here. In cases where an accident took place in the past, even years in the past, and the traumatic memory prevents us from taking that step to start riding again, **Star of Bethlehem** will help dispel it. If we find ourselves dwelling constantly on the memory, like a slow-motion replay that is painful to contemplate and causes worry and palpitations, possibly even insomnia, **White Chestnut** will allow us greater peace of mind. If we can let the Bach remedies give us that 'leg-up' when we need it, the sense of elation and joy we will experience once happily back in the saddle will ensure that we never look back.

Losing a horse

As I mentioned earlier in this chapter, for many devoted horse-owners the death of their pride and joy comes as a major shock. The Bach remedies we would choose to cushion our grief in such a case would by and large be no different from those we would choose in any inter-human bereavement. For the initial shock and ongoing grieving, **Star of Bethlehem** is a most important remedy, to which we could add **Sweet Chestnut** for the ensuing agony that may drag on for some time. As the weeks go by, if we find we cannot focus on day-to-day matters because of sad, nostalgic recollections of happier times, or we start thinking we can never be happy again, **Honeysuckle** is the remedy of choice. This might also allow us to decide to buy another horse as a replacement, which many owners find most therapeutic. And **Gorse** also treats states of sadness after losing a loved one, when there is a sense of giving up hope in anything, a sense of faithlessness.

Horse ownership gives us one responsibility that we will never have for a human being, namely the need to decide, under certain circumstances, whether to allow our loved companion to go on living or to give the order to end its life. Sometimes, when we must decide to have a horse destroyed, we can feel a terrible – though unwarranted, as we were only doing the right thing – burden of guilt. **Pine** would help release this weight, allowing us to see the truth of the matter and that it was for the best.

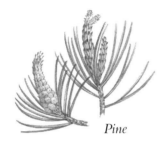

Pine

CHAPTER FIVE

BACH FLOWER REMEDIES
IN PRACTICE

Anyone wishing to use the Bach flower remedies should keep a certain selection of them in stock. Boxed sets are available, and some even come complete with an extra two bottles of Rescue Remedy. These are very useful and a good investment. However, for the purposes of treating horses and riders, certain corners could be cut to keep the initial costs down. One could start with the remedies marked with an asterisk in Chapter 2 of this book, before gradually building up the collection as experience dictates.

Remedy selection

Different people will have different methods for choosing remedies. People not as yet familiar with the system will obviously need some kind of book that they can refer to, and they might wish to flip back and forth through the pages, comparing and contrasting, writing down ideas and suggestions, until they come up with a good selection. Others use a list of the remedy names with a line or two to remind them of each one's applications. And others again are so completely expert that they can pick remedies instinctively, intuitively, without even thinking about it.

Personally, I have all my remedies lined up in a wall-mounted cabinet in the study. When I have a case in mind I walk over to the cabinet and run my eyes along the line of bottles, taking in the old familiar names and allowing the broad details of the case to flag up particular remedies. I will already have certain ones in mind, but keep an eye open for others that may interest me. Sometimes I end up with a selection of eight or nine, which I separate from the others. Then, thinking about the greater detail of the case, a process of elimination allows me to whittle the choice down to the bare essentials, the three, four, or five remedies that most perfectly fit the bill and between them form a nice tailor-made prescription for the person or animal in question.

I choose to keep the remedies in the study for two reasons. First, it is the coolest and darkest room in the house and it is where we also keep our homoeopathic remedies. But more importantly, it is a quiet place, spacious and serene with the smell of wood, leather and books, where I feel relaxed and good about the world. Why is this important?

Let us imagine for a moment that we have been thrown from our horse, or had a shock when it suddenly took off with us in fright, or that it launched a kick at us in the stable. Shaken, angry, maybe even hurt, we have come into the house to grab four remedies that we think will sort out this bad behaviour, and then we are going to march (or limp) back down to the stables and jolly well drip the stuff into the horse's water. That'll teach him…

This is completely wrong! We should always be cool, calm and objective when choosing Bach flower remedies, particularly when doing so to treat another living being. A good diagnosis cannot be made when we are in any kind of worked-up, judgemental, self-righteous state or in any other negative mental state. Hence the quiet study – we need to feel as relaxed, and as much at peace with the world as possible, when making our choice.

It is a question of attitude. We are absolutely not in the business of 'stamping out bad behaviour'. We are in the business of trying to make those around us, human or animal, happier and more able to integrate harmoniously with their environment. It must be a positive and benign thing, or else we should not be doing it. If we allow our own subjective state to colour our choice of remedies, we will almost certainly choose wrongly. In the above case, the angry rider should treat himself first with something like **Holly** or **Impatiens**, in order to reach a state where he is fit to prescribe for the horse. Indeed, many practitioners of the Bach remedies self-treat in order to remove all traces of subjective judgement from their thinking, as well as screening themselves from the negativity of what they see and hear from their patients.

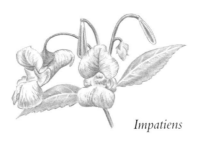

Impatiens

Dosage and practicalities for the horse

The standard procedure for treating larger animals with Bach flower remedies is to place ten drops of each chosen remedy, up to a maximum of six different ones, into the drinking water. This is wonderfully easy to do and means that you can walk away and leave the animal to its own devices. You will be sitting indoors watching TV and the animal will be treating itself!

In practice, one or two difficulties can emerge, which may call for a little thought. In most private yards with only one or two horses, water is usually given in buckets. Horses often knock these over after drinking only half the water; the solution here is to give only a little water, a third to a half of the container in question, which helps ensure that the horse will drink the remedies and not spill them all over the floor.

Where more horses are kept together, their drinking facilities are often arranged so that one communal trough serves a number of horses. This poses a problem, particularly in summer when the horses are out. So how do you make sure that the 'patient' horse gets the remedies instead of the others? Worse still, in many cases the watering facilities are of the float-regulated self-filling variety. Our ten drops will be constantly ever-more diluted, to the point that they virtually disappear! One way round this would be to isolate the horse to be treated, at least for a few hours, in a separate paddock with his own water supply, suitably laced with remedies. Alternatively, the horse could be fed the remedies on two or three sugar lumps.

To avoid spoiling the horse with too much sugar and encouraging a biting problem, chunks of carrot could be used. They are not as absorbent, but you could try making small holes in the pieces of carrot with a clean knife or other tool, and pouring the drops into them, remembering to keep the pieces level when feeding them to the horse. Only the most fickle and suspicious of horses will refuse such 'doctored' snacks!

If the horse does refuse the food, will not let himself be caught, or is unwilling to approach us, the only other alternative is to enlist some more people and move the other horses out of the paddock into another, gently keeping at bay the one you want to isolate. Place a board over the communal trough, or partition it off with a makeshift fence, and leave the horse alone with a smaller container of 'remedied' water as per usual. There is always a way round! The good news is that horses respond to the Bach remedies very quickly, so any inconvenience should not go on too long.

And for the human

When it comes to treating those of our own kind, there are also different options. If we are treating ourselves we might simply elect to take drops of the remedies neat into the mouth, straight from the 'stock' bottle. We would take two drops of each remedy, trying not to touch the dropper tube with our mouth for reasons of hygiene. Alternatively, the drops could be placed in a glass of water or fruit juice. If desired we may drop the remedies in our tea, beer or wine, without affecting their efficacy. Whichever way we do it, the two drops of each remedy should be taken four times a day at spaced-out intervals. In acute cases, e.g. **Rock Rose** for states of panic or terror, increase the dose to four drops every few minutes until relief is obtained.

Where lifestyle or the layout of the working day make it difficult to fiddle about with anything up to five or six little bottles, the ideal solution is to make up your own ready-made treatment bottle, which will be much more practical to carry about. Into a 30ml amber glass bottle with a rubber bulb and dropper tube, basically a larger version of the standard Bach bottles, which can be obtained from pharmacies, place six drops of each chosen remedy. Top up the mixture with some good-quality spring water, screw the top back on and give the bottle a good shake. Some people like to add a further teaspoon of cider vinegar for added preservative effect (if you do this, try to get hold of organic cider vinegar, which is actually very good for you and might be available at the same health store that you buy your remedies). However, this will impart a sharper taste to the liquid which some people find rather off-putting. Dr Bach used to top up his treatment bottles with a little brandy. To each his own.

Dosage from the treatment bottle should be four drops, four times daily, which again can be placed in any other drink or taken neat on the tongue. These bottles generally last about three weeks to a month.

Bach baths

Half a dozen or so drops of Bach flower remedy make a nice addition to a hot bath. Many people use this method for helping to iron out the stresses of the day and are convinced it works. Riders who are fit to drop after a long day's schooling, eventing or hacking would benefit from a soak in the bath with five or six drops each of **Olive**, **Hornbeam** and perhaps **White Chestnut** or **Impatiens** if the mind is too busy

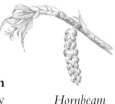

Hornbeam

working over all the memories of the day. Unlike many of the relaxing bath oils available, the remedies will leave no residue on the skin; nor will they make the bathtub greasy and difficult to clean.

When treatment fails

Nine point nine times out of ten, when Bach flower treatment seems to have no effect (assuming that the correct dosage has been properly adhered to) it is simply due to a wrong selection. Only experience can prevent mistakes from being made. It is simply a matter of re-examining the case, whether one's own or someone else's, and trying to find a different remedy or set of remedies that are better, more closely matched to the exact symptoms and underlying psychology.

When treating horses, or for that matter any animal, if your well-chosen remedy seems to fail, for instance if **Rock Rose** is less than effective in calming a very agitated and frightened horse, never ignore the possibility that there may be something physical wrong with the horse, such as severe pain caused by an attack of colic, that needs urgent veterinary attention. Serious physical problems will not go away of their own accord. Call the vet, if only for peace of mind.

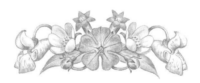

CHAPTER SIX

CASE STUDIES

Jill: A case of phobia

Mimulus, Star of Bethlehem, Gentian, Impatiens, Rock Rose, Cherry Plum

Jill, thirty-six, has had a passion for horses from an early age. As soon as she was old enough to ride, she took it up with great enthusiasm, immediately displaying a considerable talent. By her early twenties she had attained a very high standard of riding and it was the main activity in her life. In 1988, when her old horse Lucky reached a certain age, she retired him in a field behind the house and went looking for another, younger horse to buy.

She found what appeared to be a good buy, in a six-year-old, 16hh chestnut hunter. His temperament seemed just what she was looking for: calm, quiet, the ideal all-rounder that she could take out on long countryside treks. She liked him so much that she bought him immediately without insisting on a trial period.

Unfortunately for Jill, and as she later found out, the person selling the horse was in fact an unscrupulous dealer, posing as a regular owner. The horse had actually been drugged to mask its true temperament: it was highly aggressive, unpredictable, and as a vet later suggested, possibly brain-damaged. After a week or so, the effect of the drug wore off. Jill was cantering round the sand school when the horse suddenly launched her viciously into a stone wall. She was badly injured and had to be taken to hospital; and she still suffers minor lower back problems to this day.

But the main impact of the trauma was a psychological one. After that incident, she never could regain her confidence in riding. She tried repeatedly, but problem after problem kept setting her back and the months dragged into years. Riding, which had previously been such a joy to her, was now fraught with worries. A horse had only to snort or stumble, and Jill, convinced she was about to be thrown off again, would leap out of the saddle in panic. At riding schools she would insist she needed the most placid old plod they had, but even then her old fears would keep returning. Jill became very depressed, and developed many general fears and a nervousness that extended to other areas of her life and caused problems at home.

I decided on a two-tier approach to this case of fear. On the one hand there was a chronic, steady, ongoing state of fearfulness/nervousness, and on the other hand an acute panicky state that would arise when riding or about to ride. For the chronic side of things I prescribed **Mimulus**; **Star of Bethlehem**, as there was this element of a past trauma not properly dealt with; **Gentian** for Jill's despondency resulting from many setbacks; and **Impatiens** for her frustration and anger at herself for not progressing as she would have liked. As a separate prescription, in a smaller treatment bottle, she was given **Rock Rose** and **Cherry Plum** to control the panic and the impulsive desire to jump off the horse at the slightest thing. This was to be taken immediately before riding, and, if necessary, while in the saddle.

This acute prescription did Jill much good, as it showed her what she was capable of if she didn't panic. Meanwhile the other four remedies were working on her longer-term fears. Within a month she was making very good progress and enjoying riding for the first time in years. At home she was back to her old confident self, relaxed and cheerful.

Two very interesting changes additionally came over Jill. The first was this: years of feeling fearful as a result of the accident had brought back to Jill an emotional state she had suffered as a child, but which had faded as she grew older. At a young age she had witnessed violence and abuse in the household, stemming from her father who seemed to have been a Vine/Holly/Cherry Plum type of person. The chronic fear induced by her riding accident had started bringing back the same cringing, horrifying feelings and insecurities that the infant Jill had suffered then. All memories of childhood were bitter and unpleasant. But when Jill started on **Star of Bethlehem**, for the first time she started having dreams of her childhood that were not nightmarish. She remembered old friends, and good times she had had. Her problem with witnessing anger and hearing raised voices, especially those of men, subsided.

That link to the past was very much healed, once again bearing out the wonderful reputation that **Star of Bethlehem** has earned for reaching deep inside the mind to release trapped negativity.

The other unexpected side-benefit of treatment was the disappearance of her lifelong arachnophobia. The sight of a spider had always made Jill want to flee. She would not pass through a

Star of Bethlehem

doorway if there was a web overhead. But after three weeks on **Mimulus** an amazing thing happened. She was in a newsagent's buying a horse magazine, and as she took out her purse at the cash desk, there was a large spider sitting on the purse! Jill brushed it away without a thought, paid for her magazine and walked out of the shop. Only once outside did she realise what she had done! There had been no panic, no scene, no running away. The spider's presence barely even registered, and certainly not as a threat.

Jill is still riding most days, and the only remedy she occasionally uses is **Mimulus**, more as a precautionary measure than anything else. She has bought another horse, and named him Lucky II after her beloved old horse who recently passed away. All the joys of her former riding days are back with her again.

Max: An erratic jumper

Scleranthus, Chestnut Bud, Impatiens, Gentian, Hornbeam, Mimulus

This 16hh five-year-old gelding was causing problems for his rider, Mandy, who was trying to develop her skills as a show jumper. Taking the jumps at home, Max would go extremely well one minute, and then suddenly lapse into erratic and hesitant behaviour. He would approach a jump, hesitate, accelerate again and either grind to a halt just in front of the jump or wheel around and bypass it altogether. Five minutes later he would go over the same jump with no problems! His balking problem was completely random and unpredictably intermittent.

When Mandy started taking him to shows, she hoped at the back of her mind that the experience would help Max. But his problem, compounded by the added element of his and Mandy's nervousness at the show atmosphere, only grew worse. In between shows, Mandy had the help of a trainer, but the horse did not seem able to absorb the lessons he was taught. She was beginning to think that if she were to have any success with her jumping, she might have to consider trading Max in for another, perhaps slightly older and more experienced horse. She did not want to have to take this step, but the horse's antics were increasingly annoying to her and this was also detracting from her ability to concentrate on her riding. She could not understand why he was behaving this way, and often thought him stupid. One day she read about the Bach flower remedies in a health magazine.

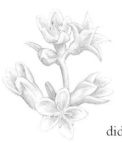

Scleranthus

Max's problem with jumping at home was obviously not down to fearfulness. I prescribed the remedy **Scleranthus** for his tendency to hesitate and be indecisive on the approach to a jump. It was the constant switching and vacillating that brought the remedy to mind. **Scleranthus** was given on its own initially, and after a few days Max's mind seemed to have settled down somewhat; he would still sometimes canter past the jump instead of going over it; but when he did decide to go over it, eight times out of ten he would go straight over without hesitation. In view of his youth and inexperience, and the way the trainer's worthy efforts appeared to 'bounce off', **Chestnut Bud** was added to the first remedy. After a further six or seven days, Max seemed better focused, less impulsive and more under Mandy's control.

At this point, though, it was clear that Mandy's own state of mind was not helping. The long period of nervousness and agitation about Max's behaviour had left her rather fraught and irritable, and setbacks would make her sigh with frustration. She was given a treatment bottle containing **Impatiens**, **Gentian** and **Hornbeam**.

The effects of these combined remedies on horse and rider had a startling effect. Max, now much more receptive to the trainer's work and less flighty in his behaviour, was a different horse; while Mandy was far better able to take things in her stride, never losing her temper, and getting vastly improved results out of Max.

Over the next six weeks, Mandy worked with Max and got to a point where she was very happy and quite confident in his ability to do well at a show. For three weeks he had not balked at a single jump and had taken everything cleanly and confidently. She decided to enter a competition and see how he went. By now she had finished her treatment bottle, and felt no need for another. However, as a precaution, she was given **Mimulus** for a week before the show. As Max's problems had always been worse when performing in public, he too was given **Mimulus**, ten drops a day in his water, starting a week before the big day.

Arriving at the show, which was about twenty miles from her home, Mandy felt no particular sense of trepidation, which was unusual for her. Max also seemed quite settled and easy-going. When it came to the jumps, it was almost as though they were at home. Only once did the horse hesitate slightly on the approach to a jump, which Mandy attributed to her own error. By and large, things went very well; Mandy and Max managed a good placing that day. For Mandy, after so many problems, it was like coming first!

Max's treatment was continued for two months, during which time they jumped at several shows. After that time, it was decided that treatment could be stopped, as Mandy felt that Max's full potential was within sight.

Chestnut Bud

Cobweb: A bereaved pony

Rock Rose, Walnut, Star of Bethlehem, Honeysuckle, Wild Rose

Cobweb, a 13hh, twenty-five-year-old grey Welsh Cob mare, is one of several rescue ponies that we have had over the years. She came to us from a sanctuary where she had lived for almost ten years. She had been very happy there, and lived a peaceful retired existence. Whilst there she had a very close companion, an older gelding with whom she had firmly bonded. All those years they lived together without any problems, until one day the gelding suddenly died of old age. When he was gone, Cobweb began to pine. She showed little or no interest in food and would stand alone in the far corner of the field they had shared, hanging her head and looking extremely pitiful.

This state of depression seemed to deepen as the weeks went by; she was losing tone and it seemed to the owners of the sanctuary that nothing could be done to restore Cobweb to her former self. They began to worry that she too might fall ill and die, and thought that perhaps a change of scenery would be the best thing for her. We agreed to have her moved to our smallholding.

On the day Cobweb was due to arrive, there was a sudden snowstorm. The conditions made driving the horsebox difficult, and it was dark by the time our transporter arrived. Our long, narrow drive was covered in deep snow and we decided it would be impossible to get the horsebox down it. So we had no choice but to walk Cobweb the three hundred yards to the house in the near-blizzard. After ten years of secure routine, the journey, the alien surroundings, and now the driving snow and howling wind were very traumatic for the little pony; she was trembling violently by the time she reached her stable. As soon as we had her under cover, she was given **Rock Rose** on some sugar, which she ate half-heartedly after much coaxing. This soothed her state of terror, the trembling rapidly subsided, and she seemed to settle reasonably well into her bed for the night.

We felt that **Walnut** would be a good remedy to help her with the sudden change in her situation and help break the link with her old life. Next morning, this was added to her water. We didn't want to give any further remedies for the moment. Better to wait and see if, as the sanctuary people had said, the change of scene would help Cobweb with her sadness over losing her friend.

Walnut did seem to have an effect in making Cobweb more relaxed during the course of the next two days, but then she began to revert to the same depressive, withdrawn behaviour that she had shown at the sanctuary. When taken out to the paddock she showed no desire to explore her new environment and would simply stand there in whatever spot we left her. In the stable, she merely picked at her food, and stood facing the corner all day long. She was quite uninterested in what went on around her, not reacting to any noises or voices.

After two more days of this we felt sure that it was not the trauma of the move to blame, but her state of bereavement. Her Bach flower prescription was as follows: **Star of Bethlehem** for sadness and sudden, traumatic loss; **Honeysuckle** for withdrawal from the present circumstances and mental retreat into daydreams, loss of hope; and **Wild Rose** as she seemed to have given in completely to her grief and had lost the will to live. We additionally decided to carry on with the **Walnut**, as this was a sensitive time for her and she must be in some turmoil. Ten drops of each remedy were placed in half-buckets of water to make sure she drank every drop; each time the bucket was filled, the remedies were again added.

A gradual change then came over the pony. First, after a day and a half, we noticed that she was no longer standing at the back of the stable with her head stuck in the corner, but was coming forward to look over the door and take notice of things around her. The next day her ears pricked up when she heard us coming, and the day after that her haynet was completely stripped bare for the first time. On the ninth day she started rumbling at us when we approached with food, and ate heartily. When turned out, she trotted to all four corners of the paddock in turn to survey the landscape before moving off to examine another part. On the tenth day we came out of the house and spied her rolling on her back and looking full of the joys of life – and we knew the remedies were really having a profound effect. Treatment was stopped at that point.

That was in the winter of 1998, and, at the time of writing, a year has passed since we acquired Cobweb. That single very short period of Bach flower treatment proved enough to completely restore Cobweb to her full potential. She gained weight and tone, her body language changed

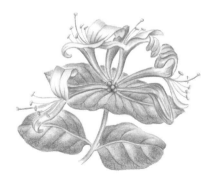

Honeysuckle

completely and she soon provided ample evidence of a very quick mind and rather mischievous ways, combined with great loyalty – as indeed befits a Welsh Cob. She has bonded well with other horses and has absolutely never looked back to that grim time when she first came trembling and snorting down the snowy driveway.

Sherman: The boisterous baby

Larch, Mimulus, Centaury, Vine, Holly, Vervain

Mike, a young businessman, was married to Annie (not their real names), a keen horsewoman. When I met her, Annie had recently bought a very large and imposing three-year-old chestnut called (quite aptly) Sherman, to whom she was utterly devoted.

Mike, whose job allowed him flexible hours, was happy to help Annie at the livery stable where Sherman was kept, and he would accompany her to shows and events; but although very supportive of his wife and full of encouragement for her, he was not truly a horse enthusiast and had little in the way of direct dealings with Sherman.

One day, Annie was called away to visit a sick relative for a few weeks. It was February, and there were all the usual tasks to attend to such as changing the horse's rugs, turning him in and out, and so on. Mike was more than happy to oblige. Annie left in the afternoon, leaving him a list of things to remember, and Mike's first duty was to bring the horse in for the night. He entered the paddock and Sherman approached him from the far side at a fast trot. As he got closer, Mike felt unnerved, thinking that the big horse was not going to stop and would plough straight into him. He stepped back and quickly climbed back through the fence.

From that moment the horse's behaviour towards Mike became increasingly brusque. He was never able to get close enough to Sherman to be able to clip a rope on him and lead him to the stable. The next time he tried, Sherman approached faster than before and the same thing happened: Mike instinctively ducked out of the way. After three attempts, Sherman was (or so Mike perceived) charging at him with ears back, and on the fourth, when Mike ventured slightly further from the fence, Sherman circled him, cutting off his exit in a very intimidating manner, then came back and headed straight for him as if to attack. At this point Mike ran for the fence, threw himself through the wooden rails and suffered minor cuts and bruises.

Mike was convinced that the horse was homicidal, and from then on

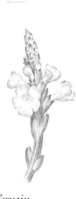

Vine

refused to go near him. He had no option but to leave the horse out that night in the rain, and when Annie telephoned him later in the evening, he was so afraid of her reaction that he lied, telling her that he had had no problems in carrying out his tasks and that her beloved horse was warm and cosy in his straw bed!

The next day, when Mike, now feeling quite desperate and additionally fraught with guilt for having lied, tried again to approach the horse, Sherman was intolerant of his presence in the paddock and barely let him through the gate. This was witnessed by a woman who kept her horse at the same livery yard and who also knew of our work with horses and the Bach flower remedies. Through her, Mike contacted us.

The first thing I did was walk calmly into the horse's paddock and approach him. As expected, he allowed me to catch him, to put a rope on him and to lead him around. He showed no signs of aggression or dominance. Clearly, Mike had adopted a submissive attitude by backing away from Sherman when the big youngster was simply expressing playful exuberance. By yielding, he had paved the way for this escalation in power-play and intimidation. Of the two, it was Mike who was the more active party and the one who could most benefit from some flower remedies.

Mike's behaviour was based on a lack of direct experience with horses, and a subsequent lack of confidence: therefore I recommended he try **Larch**. For the fear that had developed out of this tendency, I suggested **Mimulus**. And for his inability to command the respect of the horse and stand up to his games, **Centaury**. Administration was by the 30ml treatment bottle method, with six drops of each remedy topped up with mineral water, using the normal dose of four drops, four times a day.

Sherman was given the **Vine** remedy – his new-found behaviour may have started out in all innocence but it had been allowed to develop into an overt expression of a latent dominant tendency. We also chose **Holly** for aggression, and **Vervain** for his over-exuberance.

There were two weeks left before Annie was due to come home. Mike was able to find someone to look after Sherman while we waited for the remedies to show their effect on him. A few days before Annie's return, Mike was able to approach, catch and handle Sherman.

There was an unexpected benefit from the therapy. Annie, who never knew what had happened during her absence until much later, saw a subtle change in Sherman. With his tendency to exuberance he had been very headstrong and difficult to school; he now seemed much more settled and his concentration had improved. When Mike eventually told Annie of his crisis and how he had been able to solve it using the Bach remedies, Annie continued using **Vervain** periodically. As she was a very confident horsewoman, whatever dominant streak lay in Sherman remained buried when she was with him.

Vervain

Draco

Willow, Holly, Chicory, Honeysuckle, Walnut

This 14hh grey Cob pony had belonged to a farmer's daughter for eight years and she had outgrown him. During those eight years he had always had his way; his idea of being 'ridden' was to saunter down to the meadow opposite the farmhouse with the girl on his back, have his fill of grass and then come wandering home at his leisure. He was entirely his own boss and did not take kindly to any form of interference in his life. When Draco, as we named him — he had previously been known as 'the horse' — came into our hands, he suddenly discovered a world where he was expected to be ridden and he would not be in charge of his own management. He was very overweight, and, as we quickly discovered, he suffered badly from laminitis after years of unlimited grazing on a hundred acres of land. We put him on a diet and his paddock was bare and grassless, much to his displeasure.

This very proud, stubborn and wilful character soon became resentful and moody with us. One day, looking at him from a distance, I thought he had bruised his eye. In fact his eyes were black and burning like coals from his constant foul mood! He would attack any of the dogs or other horses who dared come near him; he deliberately trod on and killed two hens who had been innocently pecking around his feet. We also discovered that he had destroyed part of the fence and had found a way to get to the grass. We repaired the fence and fitted chicken wire around it to deter him. The next morning, Draco refused to eat anything at all. When he had eaten nothing for a whole day, we called the vet. The vet could find nothing wrong, and although he had never before come across a hunger-striking horse, this seemed the only possibility. The horse was so outraged at our depriving him of grass that he was wilfully depriving himself of hay. Clearly, this was a case for Dr Bach.

Draco was prescribed **Willow** for his smouldering resentment, **Holly** for his tendency towards anger and violent hostility, and **Chicory** for his sly, cunning ways and the pouting, sulky and manipulative act of hunger-striking — although thankfully he started eating again after two days, having taught us our lesson! Part of his resentment lay in the big change from his formative years of complete freedom at the farm, and so **Walnut**, the link-breaker, and **Honeysuckle** were added to the list.

Draco's negative tendencies were so deeply ingrained in him that it took longer than usual for the Bach treatment to show results. But after about twenty days he was looking calmer, the seething resentment

Willow

had gone, and he seemed to be more willing to settle into the routine. He enjoyed his restricted periods of grazing and no longer expressed his indignation when kept in the bare paddock. He began allowing the hens to scratch around at the leftovers of his hay, no longer chasing them and trying to stamp on them, and he became tolerant of the other horses. When ridden, he became much more tractable and responsive to commands. One could see that a weight had been lifted internally. A horse who had been making himself suffer by railing against his fate was able to become a better adjusted and happier horse, content with his lot in life and willing to 'go with the flow'.

Flapjack: Nervous tension in a rider

Centaury, Gentian, Agrimony, White Chestnut, Mimulus

A lady named Janet had bought Flapjack, a seventeen-year-old gelding, from her cousin who was emigrating to Australia. Janet was new to riding but had always wanted a horse, and while having lessons had been keeping her eye out for the right buy. It had to be utterly 'bombproof', safe, steady and dependable. When the offer of Flapjack came up Janet was very eager, since she had known the horse for some four years and was assured of his quiet nature.

She started riding Flapjack down quiet country lanes near her home, but quickly began to experience problems. When she mounted him, he seemed to change, suddenly becoming fearful at the slightest thing, jumping about and spooking at anything that moved. Janet's rides invariably ended with her leading the horse home on foot, feeling very dejected and unhappy.

To begin with, she thought the horse must be ill. She suspected that he might be having problems with his hearing or vision that made him feel vulnerable. However, the vet pronounced him sound. Janet continued riding, but the situation deteriorated to the point that she became afraid to take him anywhere and was confining her rides to the back garden. Even here Flapjack would play her up, refusing to walk on, helping himself to the grass, and generally behaving foolishly.

When we saw Janet riding it was obvious from her posture, stiff movements and set facial expression that she was very nervous. She admitted feeling this way, but insisted that it was a result of the horse's

Centaury

84

behaviour. We suspected that the converse was true. Flapjack was simply responding to her own lack of confidence, and a vicious circle had established itself whereby the worse the horse behaved, the more nervous Janet became, and the worse the horse behaved.

Whether riding or just handling him, Janet was unable to assert herself sufficiently over the horse. She was a very kindly person, retiring, self-effacing and somewhat shy, and she did not like to raise her voice to man or beast. Her two Labrador dogs, we observed, also walked all over her and she spoiled them endlessly. She smiled and seemed philosophical about her predicament, but something in her demeanour suggested that behind the cheerful face she was suffering from gnawing insecurities that were undermining her ability to relax and enjoy her interests. She mentioned that at night she would lie awake and churn over in her mind all the problems she had been experiencing.

Janet was somewhat surprised when told that we would like to treat her and not the horse, but was ready to try. She was given **Centaury** for her lack of authority, **Gentian** for her increasingly negative response to setbacks and disappointments, **White Chestnut** for her tendency to work things over compulsively in her thoughts, **Agrimony** for the hidden inner tension, and **Mimulus** for her developing fear of riding the horse.

After three weeks, Janet called to say that she had just ridden Flapjack down the main road to her local village, through traffic, and home again without any trouble. The horse had been perfect, his behaviour radically altered without any remedies at all! Janet's self-confidence was very much improved, and her new-found strength extended into other areas of her life. She felt more at ease with herself in general, more able to relax, and was less subject to the whims of her dogs! She has ridden Flapjack out on the road regularly ever since, and the old trouble has never resurfaced.

Chewbacca: Horrors in the past

Rescue Remedy

Chewbacca was another one of our horses, bought eight years ago by Gael in Italy. This wonderful old 15hh Argentine Creole of indeterminate age, who when standing in a paddock full of thoroughbreds looked like a mule by comparison, proved to be one of the best and most dependable horses one could wish for.

Chewbacca had had a severely traumatic past history. In the late 1980s and early 1990s, many horses were exported from Argentina to Italy. They had already had a hard life in their native country, many of them serving as Gaucho ranching horses in the prairies before being sold off to dealers for export. Eight hundred horses would be packed onto a ship bound for Italy; the voyage lasted a month and survival rate was fifty per cent. Many horses were crushed to death, and many went without food as supply was scarce and there was much fighting.

Chewbacca was one of the survivors. He then passed into the hands of a riding 'school', where horses were made to gallop up and down a beach for hours on end in the hot sun. They were badly treated, ill-fed and worked until they were fit only for dog meat. When Gael rescued him the horse was very emaciated, petrified of horses and humans alike, and on his way to the knacker's. He trusted no one, would soil himself in terror if anyone approached him, and was so claustrophobic after the horrors of the sea voyage that he could not be stabled.

Soon after acquiring Chewbacca, Gael unexpectedly had to move back to the UK and the old horse faced yet another upheaval in his life. The problem now was how to get this emotional wreck of a horse safely transported by road and sea, across Europe!

This was before Gael and I had met and before either of us had studied the Bach flower remedies in depth. But Gael had used **Rescue Remedy** in the past and now gave some to Chewbacca. Where previously he would not go anywhere near a trailer, after three days on the remedy he let himself be led up the ramp, and within a week was walking straight in. During the long journey he was repeatedly dosed with Rescue Remedy, and he was completely relaxed in his trailer, even seeming to enjoy the ride. As he passed through Customs into Britain, he was fussed and petted by officials, and did not flinch once. When he finally got to his new home, he was a different personality – confident, outgoing, and happy. For the next six years he was the ideal horse and a much-loved companion.

In retrospect, there could not have been a better Bach flower prescription for him than the combination of **Rock Rose** with **Star of Bethlehem**, which is contained in the Rescue Remedy. Terror and past trauma were his main problems, and once unblocked by the healing effect of the remedy, he never suffered again.

The St Patrick's day foal

Rescue Remedy, Star of Bethlehem, Honeysuckle, Wild Rose

On St Patrick's day, March 1999, an acquaintance who takes in rescue horses phoned us in a panic to tell us that a mare and foal had been discovered wandering along a main road in the pouring rain and brought to their sanctuary. Nobody had stepped forward to claim them, perhaps partly due to the fact that the owners would no doubt have been open to prosecution for cruelty. Both horses were in a terrible state of neglect. The mare in particular seemed not to have eaten for quite some time, and was in such a bad way that the vet deemed it necessary to have her put down. Our acquaintance was extremely concerned for the well-being of the colt foal, which was only about three months old. He was in a severely emaciated condition and now very distressed at the loss of his mother. The vet had given him an injection of vitamins and an anti-tetanus vaccination, and provided some powdered mare-milk substitute.

When we arrived at the stable yard we found the foal's condition quite a shocking sight. His ribs were protruding horribly. He had given up all hope, any will to live, and any interest in food or water, and stood forlorn in the corner of the box. It was easy enough to administer **Rescue Remedy** as a first-line treatment, as the foal allowed us to rub the liquid around his mouth and gums, too exhausted and depleted to do anything more than tremble slightly and roll his eyes.

He was given **Rescue Remedy** every half hour for three hours, until eventually his trembling stopped, he turned away from the corner of the box and accepted from us a little of the replacement mare's milk that the vet had left him. Knowing the foal would now take the milk, and having had time to watch and think about him, we dropped four drops each of **Star of Bethlehem**, **Honeysuckle** and **Wild Rose** into his bottle.

Not only did the foal survive, but in the months since he was found he has flourished. As this is written, Shamrock, as he has been named, is almost a year old. He continued on Bach flower remedies for three months, although his response to them was swift. He is very much at home at the sanctuary, and we go to visit him often.

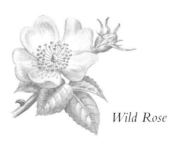

Wild Rose

CHAPTER SEVEN

HELPING OTHERS

As we move into the twenty-first century, complementary therapies are increasingly finding their place in the mainstream of public acceptance. Many people are using Bach flower remedies, homoeopathy, herbal remedies, reiki, acupuncture, aromatherapy, reflexology, and so on, who ten years ago would have thrown up their arms and dismissed all such forms of therapy as mystical nonsense.

There is much progress yet to make, but the ball is truly beginning to roll. Many practitioners of natural therapeutics across the world, ourselves included, are now being allowed access to hospitals, being asked to run courses, give talks and presentations. Many health organisations are for the first time looking seriously into applications of complementary therapies. Large corporations are giving real consideration to alternative ways of dealing with the growing problems of work-related stress and stress-related absenteeism. In Britain, local government organisations are beginning to set up new departments that will refer stressed and sick employees to complementary therapists. On the animal side, trainers, behaviourists, riding schools and boarding establishments such as kennels and catteries, are also coming to recognise the importance of such therapies as the Bach flowers. More and more vets are taking training in complementary methods and incorporating these into their practices.

Of those institutions that offer training to prospective Bach flower practitioners, the leaders in the field are the British Institute of Homoeopathy (see Useful Addresses at the back of the book), which offers a comprehensive range of courses worldwide with colleges in the UK, the USA, Canada, Australia, Germany, Japan, Pakistan, Greece and Eastern Europe, and the famous Bach Centre, which is still based in the house in Oxfordshire that was Dr Bach's last home and has carried on his teachings since his death. Practitioner courses teach the many subtle nuances of the remedies that one book alone cannot entirely capture; they also educate the student by means of real and hypothetical case studies that offer a realistic 'feel' for the sometimes difficult and complex cases they will encounter in real life.

A word of caution: practitioners intending to offer treatment for animals in the UK should be aware of the legal situation. While anyone may set up in practice advising and/or treating humans, it is currently against the law to give treatment, including Bach flower treatment, to any animal other than one's own, without the specific consent of the animal's regular veterinary surgeon. Even a fully-qualified vet with additional complementary training who wishes to give, for instance, homoeopathic or Bach flower treatment to an animal, must first have permission from another vet! Many people find these restrictions unfair and frustrating, but they are law.

On another practical legal matter, it is highly recommended that all practitioners equip themselves with some kind of third-party and malpractice insurance cover from a reputable company; a number of insurers offer specific policies covering complementary therapies of all sorts, and this can generally be obtained at reasonable cost. Even though the Bach flower remedies are one hundred per cent harmless, no responsible practitioner would even contemplate taking the risk of practising without such insurance!

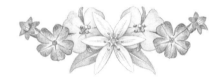

CONCLUSION

Both in concept and in use, the Bach flower remedies are unparalleled in their beautiful simplicity. That they manage to combine this virtue with safe yet highly effective curative properties, is a wonder and a tribute to the genius of their inventor. In these modern times it is so easy to equate the simple with the simplistic, even the primitive, and to overlook and dismiss that which does not involve itself with technology and the so-called 'cutting edge'. Perhaps the reason that the Bach remedies have remained in the exile of obscurity for such a long time is that they appear too simple for a society which, though slowly changing, is deeply pre-occupied with gadgetry and complexity; a somewhat cynical society, still too distanced from its natural environment, who cannot see the wood for the trees.

In fact the very simplicity of the Bach flower remedy system is what makes it so sophisticated, so very compelling, and so utterly astounding when we see its curative powers in action. Watching the way the remedies peel back the layers of negative emotion, it seems so obvious, so natural, and one is reminded of the simple wisdom that we possessed as children. It is as though we are returning to some fundamental Truth that we always knew and always held, though half-forgotten, at the back of our mind.

'It is its [the system's] simplicity, combined with its all-healing effects, that is so wonderful. No science, no knowledge, is necessary and those who obtain the greatest benefit from this God-sent gift will be those who keep it pure as it is; free from science, free from theories, for everything in nature is simple.' – Edward Bach

Useful Addresses

Ainsworths (homoeopathic pharmacy and Bach mail order)
36 New Cavendish Street, London W1M 7JH
Tel: 0171 935 5330

APACHE
(The Association for the Promotion of Animal Complementary Health Education)
Archers Wood Farm, Coppington Road, Sawtry, Huntingdon,
Cambridgeshire PE17 5XT
Tel: 07050 244196 e-mail: apache@avnet.co.uk

The British Association of Homoeopathic Veterinary Surgeons
Secretary: Chris Day, Alternative Veterinary Medical Centre, Chinham
House, Stanford-in-the-Vale, Faringdon, Oxon SN7 8NQ
Tel: 01367 710324

The British Institute of Homoeopathy (homoeopathy/Bach
courses and training)
Cygnet House, Market Square, Staines, Middlesex TW18 4RH
Tel: 01784 440467 e-mail: britinsthom@compuserve.com

British Institute of Homoeopathy worldwide:
USA: 520 Washington Blvd., Suite 423, Marina Del Rey, CA90292
Tel: (310) 577 2235 e-mail: bihus@thegrid.net
Germany: Spannskamp 2 8, 22527 Hamburg
Tel: 49 40 54767248

The Dr Edward Bach Centre (Bach information and education)
Mount Vernon, Sotwell, Wallingford, Oxon OX10 OPZ
Tel: 01491 834678

A. Nelson & Co. Ltd (homoeopathic pharmacy and Bach
distributors/mail order/information on worldwide Bach
distribution centres)
Broadheath House, 83 Parkside, London SW19 5LP
Tel: 0181 780 4200

Nelson Bach Ltd (USA Bach distributors)
100 Research Drive, Wilmington, MA01887 USA
Tel: (001) 978 988 3833

INDEX

Absent-mindedness 36

Accidents 61

Aesculus carnea – see Red chestnut

Aesculus hippocastanum see Chestnut bud, White chestnut

Aggression in humans 40; in horses 50, 59, 61, 82

Agitation 56, 78

Agrimonia eupatoria – see Agrimony

Agrimony 35, 42-3, 47, 62, 85

Aimlessness 45

Alertness 32

Alone, horses living 62-3

Anaemia 34

Anger 40

Anthropomorphism 53

Anxiety 25

Apathy 30, 34

Aspen 26-7

Assertion 28 *see also* Confidence in handler/rider

Attention-seeking 51

Bach baths 73-4

Bach flower remedies 24-52, 90; definition of 11; discovery of 20-1; dosage 72-3; for horses 14-15, 53-63; how they work 21-2; in horse world 13-14; in practice 70-4; selection of 70-1

Bach, Dr Edward 11, 17-23, 47, 88

Baths, Bach 73-4

Beech 47-8, 58, 61

Bereavement in horses 46, 79-81; in humans 30, 32, 36, 45, 68-9

Bitterness 45

Boredom 31

Boxing 56-7

Brandy 20, 73

Bucking 61

Calluna vulgaris see Heather

Carpinus betulus see Hornbeam

Castanea sativa see Sweet chestnut

Catching horse 58

Cats 37

Caution 14

Centaurium umbellatum – see Centaury

Centaury 41-2, 66, 82, 85

Ceratistigma willmottiana – see Cerato

Cerato 28, 66

Cherry plum 26, 39, 45, 51, 57, 62, 67, 76

Chestnut bud 36, 58, 59, 61, 63, 77

Chicory 39, 50-1, 59, 83

Cichorium intybus – see Chicory

Cider vinegar 73

Clematis 19, 32, 62, 65

Clematis vitalba – see Clematis

Closed-mindedness 47

Company 62

Complementary therapies 11, 88-9

Concentration 32, 36

Confidence, rider/handler's lack of 13, 28, 50, 60, 65-8, 75, 82, 85

Crab apple 43, 52
Crib-biting 62-3

Death of horse 68-9 – *see also*
  Bereavement
Defeatism 30
Depression 31, 34-5, 49, 76; in
  horses 56, 62, 79-80
Despair 19, 30, 43-7
Despondency 19, 43-7
Determination 44
Discipline 48
Disinterest 32
Dissatisfaction 47
Distraction 36
Dogs 14, 48, 54, 85
Dominance 47, 49-50, 61; in horses
  81-2
Dosage of flower remedies 72-3

Elm 46, 67
Emergencies 61
Emotional blackmail 50
Emotional imbalance 54
Emotional/mental states – *see*
  Mental/emotional states
Emotional negativity 11-13
Emotional strain 42
Emotions, horse's 55
Exhaustion 33-4

Fagus sylvatica – *see* Beech
Faithlessness 45
Falls 68
Farrier 57-8
Fatigue 33
Fear in horses 57, 85-6; in humans
  13, 19, 24-7, 60, 65, 82, 85
Foal 86-7
Frustration 31

Gentian 29-30, 35, 46, 66-8, 76, 78,
  85
Gentianella amarella – *see* Gentian
Gorse 30, 35, 56, 69
Guilt 46, 69

Habits, stress-related 62-3
Hahnemann, Samuel 18, 22
Handler 64-9; horse's reactions to
  58-9
Heather 39
Heatstroke 34
Helianthemum nummularium – *see*
  Rock rose
Herd hierarchy 65-6
Herd instinct 54
Holly 38, 40-1, 50-1, 58, 61, 67, 71,
  82-3
Home-sickness 32
Homeopathy 11, 18, 20-2, 88-9
Honey 52
Honeysuckle 32-3, 56, 63, 68, 80,
  83, 87
Hornbeam 31, 35, 73, 78
Horse, death of 68-9 – *see also*
  Bereavement
Hottonia palustris – *see* Water violet
Hyperactivity 49, 59, 61, 81-2
Hypochondria 39

Ilex aquifolium – *see* Holly
Impatience 38
Impatiens 19, 38-9, 51, 62, 67, 71,
  73, 76, 78
Impatiens glandulifera – *see* Impatiens
Indecisiveness 28-9
Insecurity 46
Insurance 89
Intolerance 47-8, 61
Iron deficiency 34

Jealousy 40, 50-1
Juglans regia see Walnut
Jumping 77-8

Lack of interest in present
  circumstances 19, 32-6
Laminitis 83
Larch 46-7, 65-7, 82
Larix decidua – *see* Larch
Leader, herd 59 – *see also* Herd
  hierarchy

Leading horse 59
Lethargy 31
Loneliness 19, 36-40, 62
Lonicera caprifolium – see
    Honeysuckle

Malus sylvestris – see Crab apple
Manic-depression 49
Memories, bad 45
Mental/emotional states of horse
    53-63; of rider/handler 11-12, 17-
    19, 64-9
Mimulus 19, 25, 56-60, 65-7, 76-8,
    82, 85
Mimulus guttatus – see Mimulus
Moods (animal) 14 – *see also*
    Mental/emotional states
Motivation 46
Muscle tension 34-5, 51 – *see also*
    Nervous tension, Nervousness,
    Tension
Mustard 35, 46, 62

Napping 60
Negativity 47
Nervous tension 13, 46, 49, 51; 35,
    67, 84-5
Nervousness in handler/rider 65,
    76-8; in horse 56 – *see also* Fear,
    Muscle tension, Nervous tension
Nosodes 18
Nostalgia 32

Oak 44
Olea europoea – see Olive
Olive 33-4, 73
Optimism 29
Ornithogalum umbellatum – see Star
    of Bethlehem
Overconcern for others' welfare 19,
    27, 47-51
Oversensitivity to ideas and
    influences 19, 40-43

Panic attacks 25-6, 51, 57, 76
Pecking-order 54, 56, 65

Personality 12-13, 21-2, 67
Pessimism 29-30
Phobias 75-7
Pine 46, 69
Pinus sylvestris – see Pine
Placebo effect 22
Populus tremula – see Aspen
Possessiveness 50
'Potentise' 18, 20
Prunus cerasifera – see Cherry plum
Punishment 55

Quercus robur – see Oak

Red chestnut 27, 47
Rescue cream 52
Rescue remedy 26, 34, 51-2, 56, 61,
    67-8
Resentment 45, 51, 83
Responsibility 46
Restlessness 36
Rider 64-9
Riding 60-1
Rigidity 48
Roads 60, 66-7
Robert the Bruce 29-30
Rock rose 24-5, 51, 56-9, 60 65,
    67-8, 73-4, 76, 79, 86
Rock water 48
Rosa canina – see Wild rose

Sadness 32, 34-5, 44
Salix vitellina – see Willow
Scleranthus 28-9, 62, 78
Scleranthus annuus – see Scleranthus
Seclusion 37
Self-confidence 41, 46, 59, 61, 85
    see also Assertiveness, Confidence
Self-control 48, 51
Self-disgust 43
Self-preoccupation 39
Sensitivity to touch 55
Serenity 35
Settling-in period, new horse's 55-6
Shock – *see* Trauma
Shoeing 57-8

Show ring 67
Shyness 28
Sinapis arvensis – *see* Mustard
Skin conditions 52
Spooking 60, 84
Star of Bethlehem 19, 33, 35, 43-4,
    47, 51; for horse 56, 58-9, 62, 80,
    86-7; for rider/handler 68, 76
Stress-related habits 62-3
Sweet chestnut 35, 45-6, 56, 68

Talkativeness 39
Temperament 17-18
Tension 62, 85
Training, horse's reactions to 58-9
Tranquillity 35, 43
Transportation 56-7
Trauma 33, 44, 51, 85-6
Tying up 58

Ulex europaeus – *see* Gorse
Ulmus procera – *see* Elm
Uncertainty 19, 28-31

Verbena officinalis – *see* Vervain
Vervain 44, 49, 59, 61-2, 82
Vexation 40
Vine 38, 49-50, 59, 61, 82
Vitis vinifera – *see* Vine
Vulnerability 41

Walnut 33, 41, 56, 79-80, 83
Water, drinking 72
Water violet 37
Weaving 62
White chestnut 34-5, 68, 73, 85
Wild oat 31, 35, 65
Wild rose 33, 62, 80, 87
Willow 45, 51, 58, 83
Worm infestation 34